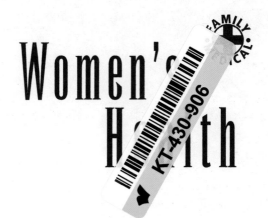

Women's Health

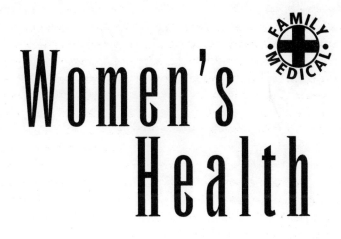

Women's Health

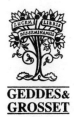

**GEDDES&
GROSSET**

Contents

A

abdominal pain *see* PELVIC AND ABDOMINAL PAIN.

abnormal presentation the occasion when a part of a baby other than the crown of its head emerges first from the BIRTH CANAL. The main kinds of abnormal presentation are BREECH, brow, shoulder, face and posterior.

abortifacient an agent that leads to termination of a pregnancy by causing a FOETUS to be expelled from the WOMB. The seaweed *Laminaria* is very effective in opening and stretching the cervical canal but does not cause uterine CONTRACTIONS. Several herbs, if eaten, cause contractions of the UTERUS and ABDOMINAL PAIN leading to ABORTION. These include blue cohosh, tansy, common rue and black cohosh, some of which are toxic in large doses. Medical abortions are carried out using natural compounds such as PROSTAGLANDINS. They can be administered as a vaginal SUPPOSITORY and trigger uterine contractions. High doses are generally required, and they can cause NAUSEA, VOMITING, DIARRHOEA and severe abdominal CRAMPS. These chemicals are effective only in pregnancies of 4–8 weeks and when used later may result in incomplete abortion with surgical procedures necessary to remove any material still in the uterus. The recently developed abortion pill is an abortifacient. RU–486 was developed in France and works by blocking PROGESTERONE, which is needed to maintain a PREGNANCY. For best results it is combined with prostaglandins, so a lower dose of RU–486 can be used. A pill of RU–486 is taken, and two days later prostaglandin is administered either as a suppository or an injection. The resulting abortion is similar to a heavy menstrual period. The drug is 95 per cent effective in inducing abortion in the first three months of pregnancy.

abortion the termination of a PREGNANCY before the FOETUS is capable of living. It may be induced by medical or surgical means or it may be spontaneous or natural, when it is usually called a MISCARRIAGE. Abortion in the former sense has been controversial for hundreds of years and is illegal in many countries. In the USA, it is governed by laws in each state, with different restrictions on how and when abortions can be carried out. In the UK, it is permitted up to 24 weeks from the woman's last menstrual period (LMP), although most procedures are carried out in the first 12 weeks of pregnancy.

There are several methods used in the UK. Prior to 12 weeks, 99 per cent of abortions are carried out using VACUUM ASPIRATION. Under a general or local anaesthetic, the cervical canal is dilated and a tube is passed into the UTERUS. The contents of the uterus are sucked out by an electric pump, and the procedure is completed in a few minutes. The woman may feel CRAMPS as the uterus contracts in size, and some bleeding is likely for around 10 days after the operation. Tampons should not be used and sex should be avoided until all bleeding has stopped to reduce the chances of INFECTION. The patient can normally go home the same day. Dilatation and curettage (D AND C) has largely been replaced by vacuum aspiration for abortions before 12 weeks. Under a general anaesthetic, the CERVIX is dilated, and the contents of the uterus are scraped out with a curette. DILATATION AND EVACUATION (D and E) is a similar method used for abortions of more than 12 weeks. The cervix is dilated, using PROSTAGLANDIN gel, and this may take 2 days if the pregnancy is 20 weeks or more. The cervix is held open by dilators and FORCEPS, and a curette and vacuum suction are used to loosen and remove the contents of the WOMB. This may take 10–50 minutes, and a hospital stay of around a day is needed. Bleeding can occur, as with vacuum aspiration. D and E has fewer complications than induction, but care still needs to be taken to avoid infection. Induction is the most common method for 12–20 week abortions. Prostaglandin or prostaglandin combinations are injected into the AMNIOTIC SAC or given by intravenous drip, and this may cause NAUSEA and DIARRHOEA. After a few hours CONTRACTIONS usually begin, following a similar pattern to full-term LABOUR by starting out as mildly painful and increasing in severity. Pain relief can be given if requested. The foetus comes out, followed by the PLACENTA, and a D and C is done to ensure the abortion is complete. The patient generally stays in hospital for a day or two, and bleeding can occur for a few days. Tampons and sex should be avoided. Induction carries an increased risk of infection so development of FEVER, sickness, excessive bleeding or vaginal discharge requires careful monitoring. Induction is a hard process both physically and emotionally as the woman must go through labour without the usual reward of a live baby. The one medical method of abortion is the abortion pill, RU–486. It can be used up to the end of the ninth week of pregnancy but is not suitable for all women. It consists of 600 mg of mifepristone, taken as a single dose. The drug works as an anti-PROGESTERONE and blocks the progesterone necessary to sustain a pregnancy. Some women react badly to the drug, which makes them sick, so the process is not effective. The patient remains at the clinic or hospital for a couple of hours to make sure that the drug does not make her sick. She is then allowed to go home and returns after 48 hours, during which time the drug softens the cervix and blocks progesterone. On the second visit a PESSARY of prostaglandin is inserted into the vagina, and it generally induces contractions and abortion within 6 hours. The patient remains at the hospital and is given pain relief if requested. If nothing happens, or there is an INCOMPLETE abortion, a D and C is carried out. If it is not needed, the patient can return home the same day (or the next day after a D and C). Some bleeding may occur for up to 14 days, during which time tampons and sex should be avoided. A check-up is done a week after the procedure to ensure that it has worked. The abortion pill has a success rate of 95 per cent.

Any abortion carries the risk of infecting the higher reproductive organs. Some women may have sexually transmitted infections such as CHLAMYDIA or GONORRHOEA without showing any symptoms, and an abortion can allow access of the disease to the UTERUS, FALLOPIAN TUBES and OVARIES. The resultant damage can cause INFERTILITY. Many women think that an abortion could reduce their FERTILITY in later life. With no infection, recent studies have shown that abortion does not normally affect fertility. Abortion is often carried out because of an abnormality detected in a foetus. The defect is normally found via AMNIOCENTESIS or CHORIONIC VILLUS SAMPLING. Termination of foetuses with genetic defects generally occurs later than most abortions, often between 16 to 20 weeks. Abortion is a complex issue with strong emotional connections. Many pregnancies that are terminated result from unprotected sex, failure of contraceptives and rape. Facing the fact of an unwanted pregnancy can raise feelings of guilt, grief and pain. These feelings are not wrong and should be dealt with and not hidden. Pre- and post-abortion counselling can help deal with the complex emotions that arise.

abruptio placentae (placental abruption) the partial or complete separation of the PLACENTA from the uterine wall. It generally occurs after the 20th week of PREGNANCY but can happen earlier. The cause is unknown, and it occurs in one in 200 pregnancies. The symptoms seen depend on the severity of placental separation and on the amount of blood loss. Blood lost from the placenta may pass through the CERVIX and VAGINA and be seen as an external HAEMORRHAGE, but it may also be retained inside the UTERUS (concealed haemorrhage) and thus hides the severity of the condition. Slight separation may result in light blood loss and is best treated with bed rest. Monitoring of the placenta and baby is carried out using ULTRASOUND. A moderate separation is when a quarter of the placenta separates and between 500–1000 mls of blood are lost. A blood transfusion is needed, and if the pregnancy is near term a CAESAREAN SECTION may be performed. Severe separation causes contraction of the uterus, tenderness, shock and possibly foetal distress. Up to 4 pints of blood may be lost, needing a rapid blood transfusion. A Caesarean section is carried out if the baby is near term, but if placental abruption occurs before the third TRIMESTER (28 to 38 weeks after CONCEPTION) then the foetus has little chance of survival. This condition is one of the most common causes of late-pregnancy haemorrhage and is more common in women who have had two or more children.

abscess an accumulation of pus in a cavity, which is surrounded by inflamed tissue. It results from acute bacterial INFECTION within a localized area. The abscess heals after it ruptures or drains and can occur internally or externally. A pelvic abscess develops inside the genital system and may arise after childbirth, surgery, ABORTION or as a result of PELVIC INFLAMMATORY DISEASE. Symptoms include pelvic pain, FEVER and chills. A severe infection results in VOMITING, very fast heartbeat, high white BLOOD cell count and a softened area develops in the pelvic region. It is treated by antibiotics, and the abscess may be drained via a plastic tube through the abdomen. (*See also* BREAST ABSCESS.)

acini milk-producing GLANDS found in the female BREAST. An acinus (or gland) is made up of glandular cells spread around a central space or lumen. The cells secrete milk into the lumen, from where it moves to a collecting duct. All the cells and ducts are surrounded by a layer of tissue with the ability to contract, which forces the milk from the collecting duct to a terminal duct for each lobe in the breast. The terminal ducts open at the surface of the NIPPLE. (*See ALSO* LET-DOWN REFLEX; BREAST-FEEDING.)

acne a common inflammatory skin disease that mainly affects the face, neck, chest and upper back. It is caused by an interaction between HORMONES, bacteria and sebum produced by the sebaceous glands in the skin. Symptoms show as comedones (pimples), pustiles (lesions filled with pus) and occasionally CYSTS. Acne is traditionally thought to develop at PUBERTY but many women have acne throughout life or it may develop in adulthood. It can develop premenstrually or may be associated with the taking or stopping of ORAL CONTRACEPTIVE PILLS. This is possibly caused by changing hormone levels. Treatment for acne depends on severity. Mild cases may be eased by washing the face with a gentle toilet soap or by drying agents such as benzoyl peroxide. Severe acne may need oral treatment with antibiotics such as tetracycline or hormone therapy such as Dianette, which also acts as a CONTRACEPTIVE.

Very severe acne can be treated using a derivative of VITAMIN A, called tretinoin or Retin-A. This cream is applied each night and takes about 3 weeks to be effective. An oral version called Roaccutane is very good against severe acne but carries serious risks of foetal abnormality during PREGNANCY. The drug is carefully monitored for any SIDE-EFFECTS in the patient but can be of considerable benefit, and the effects of treatment can last for a long time.

acupuncture a method of traditional healing that is based on the idea that disease, injury and the pain and discomfort they cause are disturbances in the body's normal flow of bioelectric energy. The pathways of this energy have been mapped as a set of more than 24 meridians, moving through over 800 points associated with specific organs and body functions. Some women find it helps PRE-MENSTRUAL TENSION, ENDOMETRIOSIS, MORNING SICKNESS and HOT FLUSHES. It is becoming more widely accepted and can treat a wide range of conditions.

acute a disease or condition that develops rapidly with severe symptoms but is short-lived in duration.

adenosis the abnormal development or enlargement of GLANDULAR tissue. More specifically, it is the presence of abnormal glandular tissue in the CERVIX or VAGINA. The condition is exceedingly rare except in daughters of women who took diethylstilbesterol (DES) during the first 3 months of PREGNANCY. This is an artificial OESTRO-GEN that was given to women to prevent MISCARRIAGE in early pregnancy and was in use until 1971. About 90 per cent of the daughters of DES mothers have adenosis, and it is believed to be a PRECANCER-OUS LESION. A form of adenocarcinoma can develop, and a careful check must be taken of all women with adenosis. A CERVICAL SMEAR TEST and PELVIC EXAMINATION should be carried out every 6 months and occasional biopsies of the vagina and cervix are recommended. A yearly COLPOSCOPY, which examines the cervix and vagina, is also beneficial. Some doctors may treat adenosis by burning, freezing or surgically removing the glandular tissue. ORAL CONTRACEPTIVE PILLS may have to be avoided as they may encourage the growth of the lesions.

adhesions bands of scar tissue that bind together two surfaces that are normally separate and that can cause pain or discomfort. They are commonly found in the abdomen as a result of surgery or IN-FLAMMATION. Adhesions in the pelvic area, involving the UTERUS, FALLOPIAN TUBES and CERVIX, or those that prevent EGGS moving from the OVARY to the Fallopian tube can cause INFERTILITY.

adjuvant therapy a type of drug therapy used in the management of certain CANCERS following on from RADIOTHERAPY or surgical removal of a primary tumour. The aim is to destroy secondary tumours where there is a risk of these occurring, and it is sometimes used in the treatment of BREAST CANCER.

adolescence the period in human development between the onset of PUBERTY and adulthood.

adrenal glands a pair of ENDOCRINE GLANDS, one on the upper surface of each kidney. Each has an outer cortex and inner medulla, both of which produce HORMONES. The medulla secretes adrenaline, and the cortex produces in excess of 30 hormones, including cortisol, corticosterone, OESTROGEN and some male hormones. The glands are stimulated by a hormone called adrenocorticotrophic hormone (ACTH), which is produced by the PITUITARY GLAND. Reduced hormone production from the adrenal glands may be linked to bone changes or OSTEOPOROSIS development in old age.

afterbirth the common name given to the PLACENTA, amnion, CHORION and BLOOD expelled from the UTERUS after childbirth.

afterpains CONTRACTIONS of the UTERUS that occur in the first few days after DELIVERY as it returns to its normal size. They tend to be strongest in nursing mothers and women who have had more than one child. They stop after a few days and may require pain relief.

agoraphobia an irrational fear of open spaces, which is normally anywhere other than the person's home. Extreme cases may mean a person is virtually a prisoner in his or her own home. On leaving familiar surroundings, a person with agoraphobia may have an ANXIETY attack with a feeling of overwhelming panic and symptoms of NAUSEA, rapid heartbeat, dizziness and sweating. Agoraphobia is more common in women and tends to develop from the late teens onwards.

AIDS (Acquired Immune Deficiency Syndrome) a disease first recognized in 1981 and caused by the Human Immunodeficiency VIRUS or HIV. Once infected with HIV, a person can expect to develop AIDS within an average of 10 years depending on their lifestyle. The HIV virus is a ribonucleic acid (RNA) retrovirus that may have arisen from a similar virus found in monkeys. Its precise origins are not known, but cases of AIDS have been identified as far back as the mid–1950s. So far two active forms have been found, HIV–1 and HIV–2, both of which cause immunodeficiency.

There are two main methods by which HIV is transmitted—by HETEROSEXUAL or HOMOSEXUAL sex and by direct 'transplantation' of the virus from one individual to another, i.e. blood-product transfusion, organ transplant and sharing needles by intravenous drug users. The virus is not transmitted through casual contact, e.g. coughs, handshakes, sneezes or kissing. HIV can be passed from a mother to her unborn baby via the PLACENTA or via blood mixing during DELIVERY. BREAST milk can also pass the virus to the baby. Overall there is a 30 per cent chance of a baby being infected if the mother has HIV. Most babies with HIV and AIDS die before the age of four. Transmission of the virus through infected blood or blood products is now largely eliminated in the developed world as all donations are tested. Blood in some developing countries may be infected as not all donations are adequately screened. Similar testing procedures are carried out on donated EGGS and SPERM in the developed countries. Formerly, some haemophiliac men were infected with HIV by blood products that were not screened, and similar accidental transmissions occurred with contaminated blood transfusions. Transmission of HIV through sexual intercourse appears to be facilitated if a woman is suffering from vaginal LESIONS caused by VAGINITIS, FIBROIDS, PELVIC INFLAMMATORY DISEASE, HERPES or THRUSH, or if she is menstruating. The use of an INTRAUTERINE DEVICE also increases the risk of infection.

At the moment the best defence against HIV and AIDS is to prevent infection by practising safe sex: use a CONDOM and spermicide for each act of SEXUAL INTERCOURSE (look for latex condoms with the BSI kitemark): use a CONDOM and spermicide for each act of SEXUAL INTERCOURSE (look for latex condoms with the BSI kitemark); avoid contact with semen, blood, faeces, URINE, vaginal fluids, etc; avoid multiple partners, especially if not known personally; avoid oral sex with a high-risk partner; use a condom if engaging in anal intercourse; don't use oil-based lubricants as they weaken condoms and make them ineffective; intravenous drug users should avoid sharing needles; sex toys or vibrators should be thoroughly washed if shared or used with a partner. These practices help to reduce the transmission of the virus through the population.

HIV causes a decline in the number of lymphocytes, called CD4+ (T4) cells, that are essential for the functioning of the IMMUNE SYSTEM, causing it to become severely weakened. As the cells are lost, symptoms appear, including enlargement of LYMPH glands, FATIGUE, night sweats, FEVERS, oral THRUSH and weight loss. Gradually the patient becomes susceptible to certain viral, fungal, bacterial, protozoal infections and tumours that are characteristic of AIDS, including PCP (*Pneumocystis carinii pneumonia*), *Cryptosporidium*, invasive *Candida*, *Cytmegalovirus* and the rare CANCERS, Kaposi's sarcoma and non-Hodgkin's lymphoma. Most people who develop AIDS die from some of these opportunistic infections within 2 years. The HIV virus can also affect the brain directly, causing a form of dementia. Unfortunately, there is no effective treatment for AIDS, and prevention is the best defence.

People are regarded as being infected with HIV if a blood test shows they have ANTIBODIES to the HIV virus. It normally takes between 6 and 12 weeks after infection for the body to start producing antibodies to the virus. This 'window period' means testing for the antibodies prior to the 3-month time lapse may generate false negative results. After infection, HIV causes no symptoms in most people until such time as they become ill with AIDS.

Women with HIV are more likely to suffer from menstrual and pelvic inflammatory disorders, persistent vaginal thrush and PRECANCEROUS changes of the CERVIX, which show that the immune system is compromised. Women with HIV should have a yearly CERVICAL SMEAR TEST because of the higher risk and refrain from smoking. Treatment of HIV and AIDS takes several forms, including trying to limit replication and proliferation of the virus. Drugs like AZT (zidovudine) were first used to treat AIDS but are now used to treat HIV infections and inhibit replication of the virus. They have some severe side-effects, including changes in blood composition, HEADACHE, sleep disturbance, ANOREXIA, NAUSEA, VOMITING and stomach pain. AZT is often used in combination with other newly developed drugs against HIV. Research is continuing into a vaccine against HIV, but progress is slow. Treatment of infections caused by HIV, such as PCP or Kaposi's sarcoma, has improved greatly in the last decade, it now being possible to treat many of these rare opportunistic diseases. Otherwise, drugs can be given to strengthen the immune response and improve its effective functioning. Many people have turned to complementary therapies, which concentrate on natural methods of strengthening the immune system, e.g. ACUPUNCTURE, homoeopathy, visualization, aromatherapy, and vitamin and mineral supplementation.

alcohol a common recreational drug taken as alcoholic drinks to relax, reduce inhibitions and increase social interaction. Women all react differently to alcohol, depending on weight, frame, height and size. They are less tolerant of alcohol than men because of smaller body size and a greater proportion of fat, so a more concentrated level of alcohol remains in the blood. Tolerance to alcohol may be even further reduced prior to MENSTRUATION. Alcohol taken into the body passes from the stomach into the bloodstream and is broken down in the liver by the enzyme alcohol dehydrogenase. In moderate amounts (2 units a day) alcohol raises the level of high density lipoproteins (HDL) in the blood, which reduces the levels of fat and CHOLESTEROL and helps prevent BLOOD CLOTS, ARTERIOSCLEROSIS and lessens the risk of HEART DISEASE. It may also help prevent high blood pressure (HYPERTENSION). In larger amounts, alcohol has negative effects. Persistent misuse of alcohol may be in the form of regular but controlled heavy intake or of alcohol dependence (alcoholism). Heavy drinking can lead to INFLAMMATION of the liver (alcoholic HEPATITIS) or liver scarring (cirrhosis of the liver). Women often develop serious liver problems sooner than men and on a lower consumption of alcohol. Excess consumption causes damage to the PANCREAS, irritation of the stomach lining or an existing stomach ulcer, and increases the risk of STROKE, hypertension and heart disease. The risks of developing CANCER of the mouth, throat, larynx and oesophagus are increased with heavy drinking, especially if a person smokes tobacco. Alcohol also acts as a depressant.

People dependent on alcohol generally feel sick, irritable and have the shakes in the morning or midway through the night and need alcohol to relieve the symptoms. They need alcohol to face the slightest STRESS and may drink alone, hiding their problem. They react angrily if someone discusses their drinking, may be aggressive, have accidents, injuries or blackouts, and possibly get into trouble at work, with the police and face financial difficulties and the loss of their families. Alcoholics are usually deficient in VITAMIN B_1 (thiamin), B_3 (niacin) and B_9 (folic acid), as alcohol increases the amounts that the body requires for normal functioning. Thus deficiency diseases, such as Wernicke's encephalopathy, can develop, and without supplementation of thiamin there can be damage to the NERVOUS SYSTEM and brain damage caused by Korsakoff's syndrome in which there is severe amnesia, disorientation and delusions. Ultimately, alcoholism can lead to a form of dementia. Sudden withdrawal from regular heavy drinking can lead to *delirium tremens*, with severe tremors, hallucinations and convulsions. This condition can be life-threatening and needs urgent medical attention and sedatives. Treatment for alcoholism usually involves detoxification (recovery from acute intoxication and medical care), counselling and PSYCHOTHERAPY to understand the problems underlying the alcoholic habit. Specialist alcohol-treatment units exist in some hospitals and clinics. Alcoholics Anonymous has a large network of self-help groups that can help alcoholics and their families.

Drinking alcohol in PREGNANCY can harm a developing baby and leave it with permanent physical or mental defects. This is particularly damaging in the early weeks of pregnancy, when many body organs and the nervous system are developing. An intake of more than 10 units a week increases the risks of delivering an underweight baby, and over 14 units a week may be linked to MISCARRIAGE. The higher the intake, the greater the likelihood of BIRTH DEFECTS such as Foetal Alcohol Syndrome (FAS). FAS results in abnormal limb development, heart defects, cleft palate and hare lip, and lower intelligence (IQ). Characteristics of this syndrome are a receding chin, an eye fold giving the look of DOWN's SYNDROME and a low and flat bridge to the nose. Development of the child may be retarded. Some doctors recommend pregnant women should not drink at all, but a safe limit appears to be 1 to 2 units of alcohol a day. (A unit of alcohol is half a pint of beer or lager, one glass of wine or one measure of spirits).

alopecia *Alopecia areata* is a disease that affects the scalp and there is sudden patchy loss of hair. A form of alopecia, called *alopecia universalis*, results in total HAIR LOSS from the scalp, eyelashes, eyebrows, armpits and pubic area. The cause of alopecia is not known, but it may be caused by ionizing radiation, ringworm, severe shingles, STRESS, chemical perming or colouring agents, and a change in HORMONE levels. Some doctors believe *Alopecia areata* is an AUTOIMMUNE DISEASE in which the IMMUNE SYSTEM attacks the hair follicles as if they were foreign cells. The disease may be linked to the ORAL CONTRACEPTIVE PILL as this blocks the body's natural PROGESTERONE and replaces it with an artificial form. There may be a hereditary link, as the disease sometimes runs in families. It may be caused by changing hormone levels after the MENOPAUSE. *Alopecia areata* can be treated with drugs such as steroid creams, dithranol or minoxidil, which may trigger hair growth. Monthly injections of corticosteroids into the bald patches are good at starting regrowth in small areas, but results can vary. The condition is usually curable, and growth returns spontaneously within 18 months. Loss of patches of hair instead of total baldness are easier to cure, but alopecia recurs in a quarter of all cases.

alpha-fetoprotein a type of protein, formed in the liver and gut of the FOETUS, that is detectable in the amniotic fluid and maternal blood. It is normally present in small amounts in the amniotic fluid, but when the foetus has a NEURAL TUBE DEFECT (SPINA BIFIDA or anencephaly), this level rises higher during the first 6 months of PREGNANCY. It can be detected by a maternal BLOOD TEST at about the 16th–18th week of pregnancy, and confirmed by AMNIOCENTESIS. If a foetus has DOWN'S SYNDROME, the level of alpha-fetoprotein may be abnormally low.

amenorrhoea (absence of periods) a failure to have periods, which may be described as primary or secondary. Primary amenorrhoea is the failure to menstruate by age 16, and the main cause is the late onset of PUBERTY. A girl may have the other signs of puberty (BREAST development, underarm and PUBIC HAIR, growth spurt) but lack periods. This may be because of a PITUITARY TUMOUR, which can be found via a skull X-RAY, or because of cryptomenorrhoea, where menstrual bleeding does occur but is held inside the VAGINA by an obstruction such as an imperforate HYMEN. Rarely, the condition may arise because parts of the female reproductive system, e.g. ovaries, UTERUS or vagina, are missing. The most common reason for primary amenorrhoea is disruption of the relationship between the ovaries and the PITUITARY GLAND. Puberty may be delayed as a girl needs to reach a CRITICAL WEIGHT before the body triggers MENSTRUATION. Many disorders can affect the pituitary, OVARY, thyroid and ADRENAL GLANDS, causing hormonal imbalance. Nutritional problems such as ANOREXIA NERVOSA or OBESITY can cause primary amenorrhoea, as can DIABETES, Crohn's disease, HEART DISEASE, tuberculosis and various drugs.

Secondary amenorrhoea occurs when a woman stops menstruating for 3 months or more after normal menstrual periods have been established but before the onset of the MENOPAUSE. The most common cause is PREGNANCY, but it may also arise because of ANOREXIA NERVOSA, excessive dieting, POLYCYSTIC OVARIAN SYNDROME, CYSTS and tumours. It can develop for the same reasons as primary amenorrhoea. It may also arise as a result of STRESS, CHRONIC diseases, e.g. thyroid disease, ANAEMIA, damage to the pituitary gland, HAEMORRHAGE in childbirth, shock, extreme weight loss and/or excessive physical activity (in athletes), and taking certain drugs, especially TRANQUILLIZERS and ANTIDEPRESSANTS. Stopping the contraceptive pill, which affects hormone production in the brain, can cause amenorrhoea for up to a year, and it may arise after childbirth and BREAST-FEEDING. Failure of the ovaries, prompting a premature menopause before the age of 40, is another cause. Occasionally the ovaries fail for a time but can become active again, restoring menstruation. Amenorrhoea is permanent after the menopause or if the uterus is removed in a HYSTERECTOMY.

amniocentesis a sample of amniotic fluid withdrawn from the UTERUS and tested to check the condition of an unborn baby. Amniotic fluid bathes the baby, and it contains foetal cells. The test is normally done in the 14th week of PREGNANCY. A hollow needle is inserted into the AMNIOTIC SAC through the abdomen, which has been numbed with a local anaesthetic. The needle is guided by the use of an ULTRASOUND scan so it does not contact the FOETUS or the PLACENTA. Around 14 mls of fluid is removed then spun in a centrifuge to separate the foetal cells from the liquid. The cells are cultured in a special nutrient medium, and it normally takes 2–5 weeks for results to become available. Tests for some metabolic disorders may take longer. Amniocentesis is not dangerous for the mother, but there is a 0.5 per cent risk that the test will trigger MISCARRIAGE. The CHROMOSOMES in the cells cultured can be tested for over 75 different genetic disorders. The test is offered to most pregnant women aged over 35 because of the increased risk of having a baby with DOWN'S SYNDROME. If one or both of the parents has a chromosomal abnormality or if a child with a chromosome defect has been born previously, the test may be recommended.

Amniocentesis can determine the sex of the foetus, its age (by measuring the maturity of the lungs), the amount of oxygen received and the chemical composition of the amniotic fluid. This can reveal metabolic disorders caused by absent or defective enzymes. The test can determine if there are structural defects of the spine, e.g. SPINA BIFIDA or anencephaly (absence of the cerebrum [brain]), and can detect the bilirubin content of the amniotic fluid. This indicates if a rhesus positive baby needs a BLOOD transfusion while inside the uterus. High acidity of the fluid may indicate foetal distress caused by a lack of oxygen. The test is very beneficial for women who carry a gene for sex-linked genetic disorders such as MUSCULAR DYSTROPHY and HAEMOPHILIA, as there is a 50 per cent chance of a male child being affected. The results can help decide if ABORTION should be considered.

Amniocentesis is also carried out later in pregnancy if the baby is to be delivered early, in order to determine lung maturity. Steroids may be given to the mother as they strengthen the lungs of the foetus, increasing its chances of survival. Careful consideration is needed before an amniocentesis test is carried out. Results are usually highly accurate and may bring relief or severe STRESS, depending on the outcome. Parents require informed and sympathetic counselling, especially if a termination is considered advisable.

amniography a special X-RAY procedure that is usually performed late in PREGNANCY to minimize harm to the baby. A particular dye is injected into the AMNIOTIC SAC and then X-rayed. The dye outlines the shape of the FOETUS clearly, and any structural defects can be detected. Because the procedure is carried out when pregnancy is well established, if a severely malformed foetus is found termination can bring emotional and physical trauma. Hence it is only used in certain circumstances. (*See also* FETOSCOPY).

amniotic sac a sac that is made from a membrane called the amnion. It forms round a fertilized EGG and surrounds the developing EMBRYO and FOETUS until birth. The sac also contains amniotic fluid, which increases in quantity from around 55ml at 12 weeks of pregnancy to 4 or 5 litres at full-term. The composition of the fluid changes throughout the PREGNANCY and may contain foetal cells that can be used for genetic testing (*see* AMNIOCENTESIS). The sac and the fluid provide a medium in which the FOETUS can move, helping to maintain an even temperature and cushioning against possible injury. During LABOUR, the sac and fluid transmit the CONTRACTIONS of the UTERUS to the CERVIX, causing it to dilate. The sac generally ruptures during the end of the first stage or early in the second stage of LABOUR, although this may occur earlier.

amniotomy a deliberate rupture of the AMNIOTIC SAC in order to induce or speed up LABOUR. Labour may begin between 1 and 8 hours after the membranes are broken, but if it does not start within 24 hours, it may be stimulated by administering OXYTOCIN, a HORMONE that triggers uterine CONTRACTIONS. The main risks are that the foetus loses the protective effect of the amniotic fluid and there is an increased likelihood of bacterial INFECTION.

anaemia a shortage of the oxygen-carrying pigment HAEMOGLOBIN in RED BLOOD CELLS. Haemoglobin is made in the body using VITAMINS B_6, B_9 (folic acid) and B_{12} (cyanocobalamin) along with iron. Each red blood cell contains 200–300 molecules of haemoglobin, so vitamin B deficiency can cause anaemia. If a woman has less than 12 g of haemoglobin per 100 mls of blood, she is considered anaemic. Symptoms include FATIGUE pallor, frequent HEADACHES, weakness, dizziness, PALPITATIONS and shortness of breath. Anaemia is common in women with a poor diet deficient in vitamins, those having heavy menstrual periods and in PREGNANCY. Blood loss from surgery or HAEMORRHAGE, BONE MARROW disease, hereditary disorders such as SICKLE-CELL ANAEMIA, and the use of oral contraceptives may cause anaemia. The best sources of dietary iron are eggs, dried fruits, liver and red meat, while folic acid is found in green leafy vegetables and seaweeds. Absorption of iron into the body is quite inefficient, but this is helped by vitamin C, which increases the uptake. Antacid medicines block iron uptake from the diet. Vitamin B_{12} is found in liver, beef, eggs, milk and milk products, and offal, but it is absorbed into the body only in the presence of an intrinsic factor produced in the stomach. If this factor is deficient, then the vitamin is not absorbed, resulting in pernicious anaemia. This affects red blood cell production and the central NERVOUS SYSTEM and is treated by injections of vitamin B_{12} vitamin every 3 months. The treatment must continue for the rest of the patient's life. Most women develop anaemia at some time in life, but it is usually easily treated.

A pregnant woman has around 3 extra pints of blood, so more of the critical vitamins are needed to make red blood cells and provide for the needs of the baby. Folic acid is required for correct development of the baby, and women with a MULTIPLE PREGNANCY are most likely to need supplements of iron and folic acid.

anaesthesia a loss of feeling that is induced by chemical agents called anaesthetics. It may affect a localized area (local anaesthetic) or the entire body with loss of consciousness (general anaesthetic). It is used to block pain from minor wounds or during surgery, dentistry and childbirth. Local and general anaesthetics are always administered by a doctor, nurse or dentist. The earliest anaesthetic used in LABOUR was chloroform, around the late 1840s. Over time, various drugs types were developed, and some, like Pentothal, acted as a general anaesthetic, which also affected the baby. In modern medicine, general anaesthesia is rarely used in childbirth. Most women have regional anaesthesia, which blocks the sensations of pain sent to the brain from a specific part of the body. These do not affect the baby and include EPIDURAL ANAESTHETIC or SPINAL ANAESTHESIA.

androgen a name give to steroid HORMONES responsible for male characteristics. The main androgen is testosterone, which is produced by the testes in the male and the ovaries and ADRENAL GLANDS in women (in very small amounts). During pregnancy, the PLACENTA converts two androgens produced by the ovaries and adrenal glands—androstenedione and dehydroisoandrosterone—into OESTROGENS.

anorexia nervosa an eating disorder in which the victim starves herself (or himself) and there is loss of at least 25 per cent of normal body weight. The term anorexia nervosa means a loss of appetite due to nervous causes. Anorexia may start in adolescence or PUBERTY but can develop in people in their twenties or thirties. It mainly affects women but an increasing number of young men are being diagnosed and children as young as eight years old are developing this condition. In anorexia the patient is often secretive about self-starvation, exercises excessively, induces VOMITING and misuses laxatives (*see* BULIMIA NERVOSA). This prompts extreme weight loss, secondary AMENORRHOEA, hyperactivity, low BLOOD PRESSURE, fear of weight gain, denial of hunger, slowed heartbeat and hypothermia (intolerance to cold). The victim may have swollen ankles, VITAMIN and mineral deficiencies and extensive growth of downy body hair (lanugo, the body's attempt to conserve heat). The body tissues begin to waste away, giving an emaciated appearance. Anorexics regard themselves as fat or obese when in reality they are vastly underweight, and may suffer from DEPRESSION and attempt SUICIDE. If anorexia persists, the sufferer starves to death.

The cause of this distressing condition appears to have a psychological basis. It may be triggered by a desire to be slim to fit the cultural ideal common in the industrialized world. It is a way for a young adolescent to control her life during a period when her position in the family and her body are undergoing change. Some people become anorexic as they subconsciously want to regress to the pre-adolescent state because of fear of developing into an adult and confusion about their sexuality. It may be triggered by a change in family circumstances, e.g. marriage, leaving home, bereavement or other suppressed grief.

Whatever the cause, treating anorexia may be difficult. The self-esteem and confidence of the sufferer need to be built up, and this can be done by family, friends and medical practitioners. Most people are treated in specialist units or in residential homes for those with eating disorders. Counselling or PSYCHOTHERAPY may help determine the basis for the condition and resolve the problem. Hospitalization may be necessary where feeding can be controlled, and force-feeding via a nasogastric tube or intravenous drip may be needed. Approximately 50 per cent of sufferers recover completely within 4 years, 25 per cent improve, and 25 per cent remain severely affected. Between 10 and 15 per cent of people with anorexia die from the condition, a proportion by suicide. Periods of prolonged starvation because of anorexia result in severe damage to several body organs and tissues, including the heart and teeth, and some of this is irreversible.

anovulatory bleeding bleeding from the VAGINA without OVULATION. In most women during the regular monthly cycle, where OESTROGEN stimulates thickening of the uterine lining (ENDOMETRIUM), there is a release of an EGG from the OVARY, and the CORPUS LUTEUM produces PROGESTERONE. The egg is either fertilized and implants in the uterine lining or the extra-uterine tissue is shed as a menstrual period. If no egg is produced, the whole cycle is disturbed. The extra-uterine tissue is lost eventually but not regularly and so MENSTRUATION becomes irregular. Anovulatory bleeding is quite common in the first few years after periods begin or in the five years prior to the MENOPAUSE. Lack of ovulation only really becomes a problem when a woman is trying to conceive. Some 20 per cent of ovulation failures are believed to result from STRESS, dietary deficiencies, OBESITY, THYROID GLAND disorders, excess ANDROGEN production and other HORMONE imbalances.

antenatal care (prenatal care) a series of check-ups, at a hospital and at a doctor's surgery, designed to monitor the physical and mental health of a pregnant woman and the development of her baby. In addition, the expectant mother (and father) receive information and advice about PREGNANCY, LABOUR, childbirth and care of the newborn infant. The checks are generally done once a month up to 28 weeks of pregnancy, once a fortnight up to 36 weeks, and are carried out every week for the last month. At the first visit, personal details and family medical history are obtained, and also the date of the last menstrual period, state of health at this stage in pregnancy and the estimated date of DELIVERY. All this information, along with examination and test results, is recorded on file and on a cooperation card. Many of the details are in an abbreviated form and can be explained by medical advisers. Ideally, the cooperation card should accompany the woman at all times in case of emergency.

Various routine tests are carried out, including height and shoe size (which help to assess the size of the PELVIS and pelvic outlet), and weight (to give an indication of the growth of the FOETUS, FLUID RETENTION or PRE-ECLAMPSIA if there is a sudden weight gain at some stage in the pregnancy). Legs may be checked for VARICOSE VEINS, ankles and hands may be looked at for the swelling and puffiness that results from OEDEMA. The BREASTS are usually examined, with the condition of the NIPPLES being noted, and the heart, lungs, eyes, hair, nails and teeth may be checked as a guide to general health. URINE TESTS may be carried out to detect urinary or kidney infections, or, if sugar, protein or ketones are present, to detect DIABETES or kidney problems. BLOOD PRESSURE is monitored, and a BLOOD TEST may be taken to disclose RHESUS BLOOD GROUP, HAEMOGLOBIN and ALPHA-FETOPROTEIN level, and the presence of ANTIBODIES to GERMAN MEASLES or AIDS. Blood may be tested to detect SYPHILIS, SICKLE-CELL ANAEMIA and THALASSAEMIA. The abdomen is examined to determine the size of the foetus, its position and the height of the top of the UTERUS (particularly valuable after the 32nd week). Foetal heart beat is checked, and an internal examination is usually carried out to confirm the pregnancy and check that the CERVIX is closed. The size of the pelvis is assessed, and a CERVICAL SMEAR TEST may be carried out. Several other tests are also utilized, some as routine and others to determine if there are specific problems with the foetus. ULTRASOUND scanning is now routine in all pregnancies to check the progress of the baby and is usually carried out at an early stage. It is also used in AMNIOCENTESIS testing, which may be done during the 14th–18th week of pregnancy. Other tests include CHORONIC VILLUS SAMPLING, UMBILICAL VEIN SAMPLING and FETOSCOPY. Together the routine and special tests all work to ensure the health of the mother and her baby.

antibody a type of protein, called immunoglobulin, that is essential to the IMMUNE SYSTEM. Antibodies are produced by cells, called B Lymphocytes, in the BONE MARROW in response to an ANTIGEN. Each antibody is specific to its antigen and reacts with it, rendering it harmless. Antibodies are responsible for IMMUNITY and are passed onto babies through BREAST milk and importantly in the colostrum. (*See also* BREAST-FEEDING.)

antidepressant a drug used to treat DEPRESSION. The majority of people suffering from depression and psychiatric problems are women. Some antidepressants are addictive and should be used carefully and under strict medical supervision.

antigen any substance that causes the formation of ANTIBODIES. Antigens are treated by the body as 'foreign' or 'invading' substances and are usually proteins. They include bacteria and viruses.

anxiety a degree of anxiety is normal at some stage in most people's lives, but it can develop into an emotional disorder characterized by feelings of fear. Women appear to suffer from anxiety (and other psychiatric disorders) more than men. The sufferer may have PANIC ATTACKS, with symptoms of increased heart and breathing rate, a rise in BLOOD PRESSURE and blood sugar level, pallor, sweating, shivering and dilated pupils. Emotional symptoms include INSOMNIA, nightmares, lack of concentration and frustration. Prolonged anxiety requires treatment with PSYCHOTHERAPY and possibly the use of TRANQUILLIZERS or ANTIDEPRESSANTS.

Apgar score a system for checking the physical condition of a baby, shortly after DELIVERY. The baby is evaluated by five signs: heart rate, respiratory effort, muscle tone, colour, and reflex response. A grade from 0 to 2 in each category is given, and the best possible score is 10. A score of 7–10 indicates a baby in good condition, 4–6 reflects a moderately compromised baby who needs resuscitation (suction and oxygen), and 3 or less is a severely compromised baby whose survival is at risk. The tests are usually done about 1 minute and 5 minutes after delivery. The system was devised by Dr Virginia Apgar in the 1950s.

apocrine glands scent glands, located in the pubic and underarm areas, that secrete an organic material with a sexually stimulating odour during SEXUAL AROUSAL. The scent is trapped by the pubic and underarm hair. Women have 75 per cent more of these glands than men, and they develop during PUBERTY. Apocrine glands are also located around the navel, LABIA minora and the NIPPLES.

appendicitis inflammation of the vermiform appendix, which, in its acute form, is the most common abdominal emergency in the western world, usually requiring appendicectomy (surgical removal of the appendix). It is most common in young people up to 20 years of age, and symptoms include abdominal pain that may move about, appetite loss, sickness and DIARRHOEA. If not treated, the appendix can become the site of an ABSCESS, or gangrenous, which eventually may result in peritonitis. This arises because infected material spreads from the burst appendix into the peritoneal cavity. Appendicectomy at an early stage is highly successful and normally results in a complete cure. Usually the pain and other symptoms become so marked that diagnosis is confirmed and action taken well before the stage when the appendix might rupture.

areola a ring of pink or brown-coloured skin surrounding the NIPPLE of the BREAST. It has nerve endings and BLOOD vessels that extend from the breast, and it contains several sebaceous glands around its edge. In PREGNANCY these glands can become more prominent and the colour may deepen. Some women develop a secondary areola as a faint coloured circle outside the true areola, and this generally fades or disappears after childbirth.

arteriosclerosis a group of diseases that are characterized by loss of elasticity, thickening and calcification of the ARTERY walls. The main diseases are arteriosclerosis, which mainly affects the smaller arteries, and atherosclerosis, in which the arteries are thickened by localized fatty accumulations called atheromas. Artheromas form at a site where there is a small area of damage to the wall of the artery. CHOLESTEROL and fats called triglycerides build up inside the wall, causing enlargement. BLOOD cells begin to collect and clot at the site, further enlarging the wall and so reducing the amount of flow through the artery. Over time this can obstruct the blood flow around the body and particularly occurs in the arteries that serve the heart and brain. An atheroma can completely block an artery, possibly leading to a heart attack or STROKE. Arteriosclerosis can begin early in life, and there may be no symptoms for many years.

Certain factors increase the risk of arteriosclerosis, including HYPERTENSION, smoking, DIABETES, high blood levels of cholesterol and triglycerides, and possibly OBESITY. The risks increase with age and if there is a family history of the disease. HEART DISEASE in women commonly develops after the menopause, often more severely than in men. Preventive measures include checks on BLOOD PRESSURE, blood cholesterol and triglyceride levels, which can help identify potential problems. Supplements of certain VITAMINS and minerals may also help as they act as antioxidants and block the harmful effects of free radicals. These can cause damage to cells and make fats rancid, and these fats are often involved in arteriosclerosis. Antioxidant vitamins and minerals include A, C, E, B_1 (thiamine), B_3 (niacin), B_5 (pantothenic acid), B_6 (pyroxidine), carotene, selenium, manganese, zinc and ubiquinone (coenzyme Q_{10}). Preventive measures include not smoking, losing weight if necessary, eating less saturated fat, which is mainly found in dairy products and meat, and being very careful to control diabetes, if present. Polyunsaturated fats derived from vegetable oils can be substituted for animal fats.

artery a blood vessel that carries blood away from the heart. An artery has thick elastic walls that expand to accommodate the blood pumped from the heart. The wall then contracts and pushes the blood along the artery, supplementing the work of the ventricles. The main disease of the arteries is ARTERIOSCLEROSIS.

arthritis the general name for a number of diseases that cause

INFLAMMATION of the joints with swelling, redness and/or tenderness. Arthritis is more common in women than men, and most forms
of the disease are CHRONIC. Septic arthritis is caused by bacterial
INFECTION in and around a joint. This is frequently caused by bacteria such as common streptococci, staphylococci, pneumococci or
gonococci (responsible for GONORRHOEA). The bacteria or VIRUSES
that cause influenza, HEPATITIS, GERMAN MEASLES or bacterial en-
docarditis can be responsible for some forms of arthritis. Rheumatic fever may cause arthritic symptoms, and this is an example
of an AUTOIMMUNE DISEASE. The most common forms of arthritis
are RHEUMATOID ARTHRITIS and OSTEOARTHRITIS.

artificial insemination a method of inserting SPERM into a woman's
VAGINA, other than through SEXUAL INTERCOURSE, so that she can
become pregnant. There are two main types—artificial insemination by partner or husband (AIP/AIH) and donor insemination
(DI). AIP is used if the man has a normal sperm count but there is
a problem with intercourse because of psychosexual difficulties,
handicap or physical injury. AIP is also done with stored sperm
from a man who requires treatment, such as CHEMOTHERAPY, that
may make him sterile. If there is a slightly low sperm count, low
volume of ejaculate or if the woman's vaginal mucus is too acid,
the sperm are placed in the upper vagina to give the best chance of
a PREGNANCY.

Donor insemination is used in cases where the woman's partner
has too little sperm, carries the gene for a genetic disease that can
be passed to his offspring, or has no live sperm. The donors are
carefully screened to check that they are fertile, have no illness or
infections such as HEPATITIS or AIDS, no family history of genetic
disease, and are mentally and emotionally stable. Most clinics try
to match the physical characteristics of the donor to those of the
woman's infertile partner. BLOOD GROUP and type, hair and eye colour, intelligence, height and complexion may all be considered. Prospective parents may wish for a donor belonging to a particular
ethnic or religious group. Donated semen is thoroughly tested for
any potential infection and then frozen until required. Insemination is timed to coincide with OVULATION in the woman, which is

deduced from temperature and menstrual charts. In some cases, ovulation may be triggered by injections of fertility drugs. The vaginal walls are held apart by a SPECULUM while the sperm are injected via the CERVIX with a small syringe or tube. Sperm may be delivered directly into the UTERUS in some cases. The woman lies down with her buttocks elevated for around 30 minutes or a CERVICAL CAP may be fitted to help the procedure. Artificial insemination is generally carrried out on the 12th and 14th day of a 28–day MENSTRUAL CYCLE for about 4 months. The pregnancy rate with fresh semen is 60–70 per cent; with frozen semen it is approximately 55 per cent. Women with a history of pelvic disease, disorders of ovulation or ENDOMETRIOSIS, and those aged over 30 have a lower success rate with artificial insemination.

assisted conception CONCEPTION of a FOETUS by IN VITRO FERTILIZATION.

asymptomatic a name given to a disease that shows no outward symptoms. Diseases such as PELVIC INFLAMMATORY DISEASE or TRICHOMONAS are often present but with no physical symptoms.

autoimmune disease a set of disorders in which the body attacks itself by manufacturing ANTIBODIES against normal tissue. Examples include RHEUMATOID ARTHRITIS, MULTIPLE SCLEROSIS, MYASTHENIA GRAVIS, pernicious ANAEMIA, SYSTEMIC LUPUS ERYTHEMATOSUS and several forms of thyroid disorder including GRAVES' DISEASE. The cause of autoimmune diseases is not known, but they are far more prevalent in women. This may be related to the fact that women support the growth of foreign tissue (the FOETUS) in PREGNANCY, requiring the production of specialized substances to suppress the immune responses.

B

back pain the spine is made up of approximately 30 vertebrae and between each pair there is a cartilaginous disc. The discs and vertebrae are held together with ligaments, and most causes of mild back pain occur because of twisting or stretching of these structures.

Back pain is very common in both men and women, and it can be caused by various factors. Poor posture and hence muscle tension give rise to 90 per cent of cases of back pain. This results from poor seating in chairs that do not give sufficient support and is a common problem at work, in the home or car. It is also caused by bending and lifting incorrectly or by a repetitive strain. There may be disorders affecting the discs between the bones, the most common being a 'slipped' disc, in which it ruptures or moves out slightly from between the vertebrae. This commonly occurs if a person bends or twists suddenly and can be very painful. Emotional STRESS, kidney INFECTION, OSTEOARTHRITIS, OSTEOPOROSIS and pelvic PROLAPSE can all be a cause of back pain. OBESITY strains the back and can lead to discomfort, and women are particularly prone to back problems from gynaecological causes. Conditions such as OVARIAN CYSTS, FIBROIDS, infection of the FALLOPIAN TUBES, ENDOMETRIOSIS, PREGNANCY and LABOUR may produce severe back pain. It may be eased by physiotherapy, osteopathy, chiropractic, ACUPUNCTURE or shiatsu (a form of massage) and by treatment of the underlying cause. Preventive methods, include correct lifting, good posture and avoidance of actions that cause strain.

barrier method a method of CONTRACEPTION that physically prevents the SPERM from reaching the EGG. They include the CERVICAL CAP, DIAPHRAGM, CONTRACEPTIVE SPONGE and male and female CONDOM. Some SPERMICIDES render sperm inactive so that they cannot reach the egg. These methods have varying success rates in preventing PREGNANCY, and most can also protect against various SEXUALLY TRANSMITTED DISEASES, including AIDS.

Bartholin's glands a pair of GLANDS found on each side of the vaginal entrance that open into the VAGINA. They are thought to secrete small quantities of mucus that lubricate the vagina during SEXUAL AROUSAL and intercourse. They may become infected by bacteria (such as gonococci, which cause GONORRHOEA), and these infections require treatment with antibiotics and possibly surgery.

basal body temperature the lowest temperature of a normal healthy person during waking hours. During the MENSTRUAL CYCLE, a drop in temperature usually happens 12–24 hours before OVULATION, and it then rises again because of the action of the hormone PROGES-TERONE. Thus a record of the basal body temperature is of value in the timing of BIRTH CONTROL and CONCEPTION. It may be affected by FATIGUE, emotional STRESS, an INFECTION, or other factors. Some women do not have a clear pattern of basal body temperature even if they ovulate regularly.

basal metabolism the minimum amount of energy that is utilized by the body to maintain vital processes such as respiration, BLOOD circulation and digestion. Factors such as age, thyroid activity and sex affect basal metabolic rate. (*See also* METABOLISM.)

benign a term normally applied to a TUMOUR that is not cancerous and does not invade the tissue where it develops or spread to other sites in the body. (*See also* MALIGNANT.)

biopsy a minor operation in which a sample of body tissue is removed for examination, normally carried out to detect a disease or abnormality. Various methods are used, including a scrape to remove surface cells, a needle to drain fluid, a hollow needle to remove samples of tissue from an organ such as the liver, fibre-optic excision and surgical techniques. The technique used depends on the tissue that is to be examined, and methods such as MAMMOGRA-PHY, X-RAYS and ULTRASOUND are used to locate and guide sampling of the suspect tissue.

birth canal the passage from the UTERUS through the VAGINA, down which a baby passes during childbirth.

birth control a term for any device, method or substance used to prevent PREGNANCY. The name was invented by Margaret Sanger in the USA, who fought to improve the availability of birth control, despite several state laws against CONTRACEPTION, and to disseminate information. Many methods have been tried since ancient times, including placing material such as honey, silk, paper, serpent fat and lemon juice inside the VAGINA to prevent CONCEPTION. Today, a variety of contraceptive methods are available (*see* CONDOM, DIAPHRAGM, CERVICAL CAP, DOUCHING, NATURAL FAMILY PLANNING, MINI-PILL, ORAL CONTRACEPTIVE PILL, SPERMICIDES, COITUS INTERRUP-TUS).

birth defects physical abnormalities present in children at birth that may or may not be hereditary. Birth defects can arise from two sources—external influences, i.e. the mother's exposure to VIRUS IN-FECTION, various CHRONIC diseases, drugs (including nicotine and ALCOHOL), radiation, malnutrition, and damage to the baby during LABOUR and DELIVERY. The other is genetic abnormalities in GENES or CHROMOSOMES, which may be called genetic disorders. These disorders may be dominant or recessive. However most recessive genes are masked by the presence of a normal dominant counterpart. If both parents carry an abnormal recessive gene then the child has a 1 in 4 chance of having the disorder or a 2 in 4 chance of being a carrier. The most common dominant disorder is familial hypercholesterolaemia, in which the BLOOD CHOLESTEROL levels are so elevated that there is a risk of heart attack and narrowing of the arteries. This affects 1 in 500 people, and all babies are tested for its presence. Recessive disorders number about 950, and the most common are CYSTIC FIBROSIS, SICKLE-CELL ANAEMIA, THALASSAEMIA and TAY-SACHS DISEASE.

There are three kinds of genetic disorder—chromosome defects, single gene disorders, and polygenic or multifactorial disorders. Chromosome disorders involve either a lack or an excess of DNA, which results in structural defects or changes to the normal number of chromosomes. The most common disorder is DOWN'S SYNDROME, where the child has an extra chromosome No. 21. Certain chromosome defects affect the X and Y sex chromosomes, and these produce children with obscure sexuality. Males suffer from KLINEFEL-TER'S SYNDROME, in which there are three sex chromosomes, XXY, and females have TURNER'S SYNDROME, in which there is only one X-CHROMOSOME.

Single-gene disorders occur when there are 1 or 2 mutant genes that differ from the normal one. If the gene is dominant there is a 50 per cent chance the child will have the disorder. Over 1200 dominant-gene defects have been found, including Huntington's chorea (a progressive neurological disorder that is eventually fatal) and familial hypercholesterolaemia. Recessive single-gene defects have been mentioned earlier, and there is a 25 per cent chance of a baby having the disorder if both parents carry the gene. Polygenic disorders arise because pairs of genes interact and they are affected by external factors.

These defects include cleft palate, hare lip, club foot and SPINA BIFIDA. These disorders may be related to maternal deficiency in certain VITAMINS and minerals, e.g. folic acid, (vitamin B9). Several disorders occur only on the X-chromosome and are recessive. Thus, a female who has one normal X-chromosome and one that is defective will not have a disorder but is a carrier of the abnormality. Since men have a Y-CHROMOSOME, they inherit the disorder as the Y-chromosome cannot mask the defective X-chromosome. HAEMOPHILIA, MUSCULAR DYSTROPHY and fragile X-syndrome (which leads to a form of mental retardation) are examples of these gender-linked diseases. Many of these genetic defects can be tested for early in PREGNANCY, and an affected FOETUS can be aborted if it is deemed advisable. GENETIC COUNSELLING and SCREENING are helpful in determining if either parent carries a gene for a particular genetic disorder and can reduce the number of affected children born. (*See also* AMNIOCENTESIS; CHORIONIC VILLUS SAMPLING; CONGENITAL DEFECT; FETOSCOPY; GAUCHER'S DISEASE; PHENYLKETONURIA; THALASSAEMIA.)

birthing room a hospital room where LABOUR, DELIVERY and recovery takes place. It is designed to be comfortable and like home so it helps the mother to relax, lessens fears and eases tension. It often has easy chairs, cushions, music and soft lighting, and close friends or children may be permitted to stay with the mother during the birth if she wishes. The room may contain standard equipment for monitoring the FOETUS and oxygen, etc. It is an intermediate option between a HOME BIRTH and a clinical hospital delivery.

birthmark a blemish or area of pigmentation found on the skin. They are brown, pink, purple or red in colour and are generally caused by a collection of BLOOD vessels below the skin. There are various types, including stork bites (pink patches on the eyelids or nose that disappear after about a year). Mongolian spots are blue marks found on the lower back, particularly on black, Asian or Mediterranean babies. Strawberry birthmarks are red and vary in size, and port-wine stains are large red or purple marks often found on the face and neck. They are permanent but can be removed in later life by laser treatment.

birth weight the weight of a newborn baby, which is directly related to its maturity and chances of survival. Average birth weight is 2.5–4.5 kilograms (5lb 8oz–9lb 12oz). Low birth weight babies may be PREMATURE, have a genetic disorder or be malnourished. Malnutrition may be caused by disease in the mother, such as HYPERTENSION, DIABETES or kidney disorders.

bisexual a person who desires and/or engages in both HETEROSEXUAL and HOMOSEXUAL intercourse.

bladder a sac of fibrous and muscular tissue in the front of the PELVIS that acts as a reservoir for URINE. Urine enters the bladder through the URETERS leading from the kidneys and is eliminated through the URETHRA. The female bladder is very prone to INFECTION or INFLAMMATION from bacteria in the urethra. The muscles of the pelvic floor support the bladder, VAGINA and RECTUM, and these can be weakened by PREGNANCY and childbirth, resulting in CYSTOCELE. (*See also* CYSTITIS; STRESS INCONTINENCE.)

bleeding, vaginal normally this is MENSTRUAL FLOW but some disruption of the MENSTRUAL CYCLE can cause BREAKTHROUGH BLEEDING. The flow is derived from the UTERUS and is lost through the VAGINA. Any bleeding from the vagina before MENARCHE and after MENOPAUSE should be investigated promptly as it may indicate the presence of a serious disease such as CANCER. Vaginal bleeding during PREGNANCY is also a cause for concern and should be investigated promptly. Vaginal bleeding may be caused by hormonal changes and failure to ovulate, ECTOPIC PREGNANCY, MISCARRIAGE, or disease affecting the pelvic organs including OVARIAN CYSTS, FIBROIDS or an endometrial POLYP. The use of contraceptive pills or an INTRAUTERINE DEVICE are other causes. If bleeding occurs after SEXUAL INTERCOURSE then it may be a CERVICAL EVERSION that is causing the problem. Treatment depends upon the cause and further investigation such as a D AND C may be required. (*See also* ANOVULATORY BLEEDING; HAEMORRHAGE; POSTMENOPAUSAL BLEEDING; POSTPARTUM HAEMORRHAGE.)

blood a suspension of RED BLOOD CELLS (or corpuscles), white blood cells (leucocytes) and platelets (small disc-shaped cells involved in BLOOD CLOTting) in a liquid medium, blood plasma. The circulation of blood through the body provides a mechanism for transporting substances. Its functions include: (1) carrying oxygenated blood from the heart to all tissues via the arteries while the VEINS return deoxygenated blood to the heart; (2) carrying essential nutrients, e.g. glucose, fats and amino acids, to all parts of the body; (3) removing the waste products of METABOLISM—ammonia and carbon dioxide—to the liver where urea is formed and then transported by the blood to the kidneys for excretion; (4) carrying important molecules, e.g. HORMONES, to their target cells.

The red blood cells, produced in the BONE MARROW, are HAEMO-GLOBIN-containing discs while the white varieties vary in shape and are produced in the marrow and lymphoid tissue. The plasma comprises water, proteins and electrolytes, and forms approximately half the blood volume.

blood clot a hard mass of BLOOD platelets, trapped RED BLOOD CELLS and fibrin. After tissue damage, blood vessels in the area are constricted and a plug forms to seal the injured part. The plug formation is initiated by an enzyme released by the damaged blood vessels and platelets.

blood count or **complete blood count** (CBC) a count of the red and white blood cells per unit volume of BLOOD. The count may be performed manually, using a microscope, or electronically.

blood groups the division and classification of people into one of four main groups based on the presence of ANTIGENS on the surface of the RED BLOOD CELLS (corpuscles). The classifying reaction depends on the serum of one person's BLOOD agglutinating (clumping together) the red blood cells of someone else. The antigens, known as agglutinogens, react with ANTIBODIES (agglutinins) in the serum. There are two agglutinogens, termed A and B, and two agglutinins, called anti-A and anti-B. This gives rise to four groups: corpuscles with no agglutinogens, group O; with A; with B; and with both A and B (hence blood group AB). The agglutinin groups match those of the agglutinogens, thus a person of blood group B has anti-A serum in his or her blood. It is vital that blood groups are matched

for transfusion because incompatibility will produce BLOOD CLOT-
ting.

The RHESUS FACTOR (Rh factor) is another antigen (named after
the rhesus monkey, which has a similar antigen), those with it being Rh positive and those without Rh negative. About 85 per cent
of people are Rh-positive. If a Rh-negative person receives Rh-
positive blood, or if a Rh-positive foetus is exposed to antibodies
to the factor in the blood of its Rh-negative mother, then haemolysis occurs in the FOETUS and newborn child. This may cause the
STILLBIRTH of the child or JAUNDICE after birth. Testing of pregnant
women is thus essential.

blood pressure the pressure of the BLOOD on the heart and blood
vessels in the system of circulation. Also, the pressure that has to
be applied to an ARTERY to stop the pulse beyond the pressure point.
Blood pressure peaks at a heartbeat (systole) and falls in between
(diastole). The systolic pressure in young adults is equivalent to
approximately 120 mm mercury (and 70 mm in diastole). The pressure also depends on the hardness and thickness of vessel walls,
and blood pressure tends to increase with age as arteries thicken
and harden. A temporary rise in blood pressure may be precipitated by exposure to cold; a permanent rise by kidney disease and
other disorders. A lower blood pressure can be induced by a hot
bath or caused by exhaustion. The instrument used to measure
blood pressure is the sphygmomanometer.

blood tests a testing of a sample of BLOOD for disease or other abnormality. The most common blood test is for ANAEMIA, measuring
the level of HAEMOGLOBIN or the percentage of RED BLOOD CELLS.
Blood serum is the part of the blood without any blood cells or
blood coagulation factors, and it is often examined to detect and
identify ANTIBODIES. Serum tests for CHOLESTEROL, blood sugar,
triglycerides and minerals (e.g. potassium) are done to determine
the presence of disease or deficiency. The levels of blood urea ni-
trogen, creatinine, various enzymes, uric acid, proteins, calcium and
phosphorus in blood can indicate how effectively the body is functioning and if any disease is present. During PREGNANCY, various
blood tests are carried out. At 16 weeks a test for ALPHA-FETOPROTEIN

(a protein produced by the embryo yolk sac and then the foetal liver in varying quantites) is carried out. Elevated levels of alpha-fetoprotein occur in multiple pregnancies or may indicate an error in the expected date of DELIVERY. It may also indicate a threat of MISCARRIAGE or that there are abnormalities in the baby's digestive tract or kidneys. An unusually low level of alpha-fetoprotein may suggest that the foetus has DOWN'S SYNDROME. (*See also* BLOOD COUNT.)

bonding the process by which a close emotional relationship is established between a newborn baby and its parents. The bond formed at the beginning of life has a long-lasting effect on the parent/child relationship. The baby can differentiate voices before it is born, and both mother and father are now encouraged to talk to their baby while it is still in the UTERUS. Babies can recognize pieces of music that have been played to them before birth, and they know the sound of the mother's heartbeat. Just after the baby has been born and checked by the medical team, the mother should hold and cuddle her infant next to her skin. It is a good idea to put the baby to the BREAST, even if it does not want to feed, as this aids bonding and stimulates the delivery of the PLACENTA. The baby gets used to the smell of its mother's skin, and smiling and talking to the child helps recognition. The father should be allowed to cuddle and hold his baby within half an hour of DELIVERY if at all possible. Fathers can bond to their children just as strongly as mothers. Later on, holding the baby firmly but gently and having skin-to-skin contact will help associate both parents with loving, caring and security. Evidence shows that the more physical contact a baby has, the happier and healthier it becomes.

Obviously, bonding may not be instantaneous and not all newborns fulfil the parents prebirth ideal. PREMATURE babies may look red with wrinkled skin as they do not have the layers of fat that are normally laid down in the final weeks of PREGNANCY. It can be difficult to relate to the baby, and medical staff generally encourage parents to touch and stroke premature babies whenever possible. Special equipment such as incubators and monitors may be intimidating, but studies show that premature babies breathe more readily if they are stroked and spoken to in a loving manner. Once a baby is breathing on its own, contact becomes more natural. Bonding in the early stages takes time and does not need to be rushed. A mother may require time to recover from the physical and emotional trauma of birth. There are no set rules and the baby benefits considerably from interaction with both its parents.

bone the hard connective tissue that with cartilage forms the skeleton. Bone has a matrix of collagen fibres with bone salts (crystalline calcium phosphate or hydroxyapatite, in which are the bone cells, osteoblasts and osteocytes). The bone cells form the matrix. There are two types of bone: compact or dense, forming the shafts of long bones; and spongy or cancellous, which occurs on the inside and at the ends of long bones and also forms the short bones. Compact bone is a hard tube covered by the periosteum (a membrane) and enclosing the marrow and contains very fine canals around which the bone is structured in circular plates. (*See also* BONE MARROW.)

bone marrow a soft tissue found in the spaces of BONES. In young animals all bone marrow, the red marrow, produces BLOOD cells. In older animals the marrow in long bones is replaced by yellow marrow, which contains a large amount of fat and does not produce blood cells. In mature animals the red marrow occurs in the ribs, sternum, vertebrae and the ends of the long bones (e.g. the femur). The red marrow contains myeloid tissue with erythroblasts from which RED BLOOD CELLS develop. Leucocytes (a type of white blood cell) also form from the myeloid tissue and themselves give rise to other cell types.

Braxton-Hick contractions weak, irregular CONTRACTIONS of the UTERUS that occur during PREGNANCY. They occur from about 32 weeks onwards but may be noticeable only in the last few weeks. The abdomen may become tense and firm periodically, and they contribute to the EFFACEMENT and dilation of the CERVIX. They are not normally painful but may be uncomfortable for some women. Sometimes they are strong enough to be mistaken for true LABOUR. (*See also* FALSE LABOUR.)

breakthrough bleeding bleeding from the VAGINA that occurs between menstrual periods and commonly happens around the time of OVULATION, causing no harm. (*See also* BLEEDING, VAGINAL.)

breast a pair of glands, the mammary glands, that produce milk. Each gland is composed of milk lobules that produce the milk, and these are embedded in fatty tissue. The milk travels from lobules into ducts, and these unite to form larger ducts and reservoir structures called ampullae. Each large duct discharges milk through a separate opening in the nipple. The breast is richly supplied with BLOOD and LYMPH vessels. The breast usually extends from the 2nd or 3rd rib down to the 5th or 6th, and it is underlaid by the pectoral muscles. A tail of breast tissue extends into the armpit.

The female breast starts to form in the FOETUS at around 6 weeks' GESTATION, and both males and females develop NIPPLES. In females, the milk ducts begin to form and they open up on to the nipple at 12 weeks' gestation. No more development occurs until PUBERTY, when OESTROGEN stimulates the milk ducts to lengthen and increase in number by branching. As these ducts develop, the AREOLA starts to form and becomes pigmented. Connective and fatty tissue forms, and PROGESTERONE causes the milk-producing GLANDS at the ends of the milk ducts to develop. The development of milk lobules in the breast continues until about age 25.

Female breast development is an important secondary sexual characteristic. The size and shape of the breasts is governed by various factors, including fat deposits, NUTRITION, heredity, the effects of oestrogen and progesterone, the strength of the supporting ligaments and WEIGHT GAIN or loss. Additional support can be provided by a well-fitting bra. The breasts are susceptible to a range of disorders. (*See also* ACINI; BREAST CANCER; BREAST CYST; BREAST-FEEDING; BREAST PLASTIC SURGERY; BREAST SELF-EXAMINATION; CYSTIC MASTITIS; FIBROADENOMA; GALACTOCELE; GALACTORRHOEA; INTRADUCTAL PAPILLOMA; INVERTED NIPPLE; LACTATION; LET-DOWN REFLEX; MAMMARY DUCT ECTASIA; MAMMOGRAPHY; MASTALGIA; MASTECTOMY; MASTITIS; NIPPLE DISCHARGE; NIPPLE RETRACTION; PHYLLODES TUMOUR; SCLEROSING ADENOSIS.)

breast abscess a BREAST abscess can develop during BREAST-FEEDING if the NIPPLES become dry and cracked as bacteria enter the fissures and the affected area becomes red, swollen and tender to touch. The patient may experience FEVERS and chills, and a large hard lump develops. Hot or cold compresses may be used to ease the pain. The abscess is treated with antibiotics and may be drained when ripe. These problems were formerly very common, particularly after a first baby, but early antibiotic treatment normally cures the INFECTION before an ABSCESS forms.

breast cancer the development of abnormal cells in the BREAST tissue, forming a lump or tumour. This is the most common type of CANCER in women, and there are at least 15 different kinds, depending on the site of development. All have different rates of growth and varying tendencies to metastasize (spread to other areas). Breast cancer is a MALIGNANT growth of tissue that affects approximately 26,000 women a year in the UK. It is normally found when a suspicious lump is detected, but 90 per cent of all breast lumps are BENIGN. Other signs of cancer are a change in breast size or shape, a swelling in the armpit or upper arm, NIPPLE RETRACTION, thickening, dimpling or ulceration of the skin, and a lump on the NIPPLE.

Women are recommended to examine their breasts once a month to detect any changes or lumps. If BREAST SELF-EXAMINATION detects a lump, the family doctor should be consulted, who will normally refer the woman to a hospital clinic for further investigation. MAMMOGRAPHY to locate the lump or ULTRASOUND examination may be carried out. THERMOGRAPHY can also locate a cancer nodule as it is hotter than surrounding tissue. If a lump is confirmed, it needs to be examined by draining some cells from it via a needle (needle aspiration), BIOPSY or surgical removal. The tissue removed is tested for cancer and, if positive, treatment begins as soon as possible. Further tests will be done to establish if the cancer has spread—possibly including BONE and liver scans. This helps to determine the stage of development of the cancer, which affects the course of treatment. Current convention means that breast cancer is usually treated surgically along with CHEMOTHERAPY, RADIOTHERAPY and HORMONE therapy. Surgery used to involve the removal of the whole breast, but this is less common today. Techniques of lumpectomy or segmentectomy remove the breast lump

and some surrounding tissue, with follow-up radiotherapy. MAS-
TECTOMY (removal of the breast) may still be necessary if the lump
is not easily accessible, and some women prefer this so that the
disease cannot recur. Radiotherapy kills any remaining cancer cells
using gamma radiation or X-RAYS. Chemotherapy uses CYTOTOXIC
drugs to kill cancer cells both in the breast and elsewhere in the
body. Hormone therapy may be used, as OESTROGEN and PROGES-
TERONE influence all breast cells, including cancerous ones. However, many cancers are hormone-dependent. Oestrogen promotes
growth of cancer cells, so it may be advisable to stop the production of oestrogen. This used to be done by surgically removing the
ovaries, ADRENAL GLANDS or PITUITARY GLAND, but today certain
drugs are given instead. Modern treatments have greatly improved
the quality and quantity of life for breast cancer patients. In many
cases, the disease can be cured, and survival times are
increasing.Women should not regard DIAGNOSIS of breast cancer as
an automatic death sentence. Many try complementary therapy in
the form of VITAMIN and mineral supplements, ACUPUNCTURE,
aromatherapy, reflexology, healing, massage, homoeopathy, counselling, visualization, deep relaxation techniques and meditation.
These may help lessen the SIDE-EFFECTS of chemotherapy or radiotherapy, aid recovery and help provide a positive boost to self-confidence. Breast cancer has severe mental and emotional effects on a
woman and her partner. Many women are now treated in specialist
cancer units, where surgeons have more experience of treating the
disease and specialist breast-care nurses offer support and advice
from diagnosis onwards. There are also many self-help groups that
offer help and support.

Some women are more at risk of developing breast cancer. The
disease sometimes seems to run in families, and two GENES linked
to breast cancer have been discovered in recent years. For women
at risk of developing the disease, tamoxifen may be given as this is
an anti-oestrogen and can reduce the chances of cancer developing. Women with a previous history of benign breast lumps, those
who have not borne children, those aged over 40 and white are all
at greater risk. A high-fat, high-protein and low-carbohydrate diet,

which is common in industrialized countries, may increase the risk, but BREAST-FEEDING appears to protect against this disease. This effect can be mimicked by nipple stimulation, which some doctors believe aids prevention by encouraging the production of certain natural hormones. A diet rich in antioxidant vitamins and minerals can help prevent cell damage by carcinogens and free radicals. (*See also* PAGET'S DISEASE OF THE NIPPLE; INFLAMMATORY BREAST CANCER.)

breast cysts accumulations of fluid that form in a duct or lobule of the BREAST tissue. They are most common in women aged between 35 and 55 in whom levels of HORMONES are fairly high. A cyst can be up to 5 cm in diameter and may be felt as a hard lump. Leakage of fluid from a CYST into surrounding tissue can cause great pain. Cysts are treated by aspirating the fluid through a needle, and this is then examined. Recurrence is an uncommon problem, and they can be treated with hormonal drugs, if necessary.

breast-feeding the suckling of an infant and the natural method of feeding in mammals and humans. Most authorities believe that it is the best way of providing nourishment for a baby as the milk contains all the nutrients required in an easily digestible form, as well as ANTIBODIES to protect against INFECTION and allergies. Since breast-feeding is regulated by the baby, over-feeding and early OBESITY is unlikely, and the milk is always warm, sterile, fresh and available. The fluid produced in the first few days after childbirth is called colostrum, and it is protein-rich, containing antibodies and a natural laxative to stimulate the baby's bowels. Milk production begins 3–5 days after childbirth, and is triggered by hormonal changes. Suckling stimulates the nerve endings in the AREOLA and the production of PROLACTIN and OXYTOCIN hormones from the pituitary gland. Prolactin stimulates the production of milk while oxytocin plays a part in the LET-DOWN REFLEX, in which the muscle fibres surrounding the milk glands contract, moving milk to the milk ducts. Oxytocin also helps the UTERUS return to normal size after childbirth. Breast-feeding helps the mother lose the extra weight gained during PREGNANCY but does not appear to have any permanent effect on the size and shape of the BREASTS and lessens the risk of developing BREAST CANCER in later life. Women who have had breast reconstruction surgery with silicone implants and breast augmentation may still be able to breast-feed. Women who have had reduction surgery may not be able to breast-feed if too much secretory tissue has been removed or too many mammary ducts have been cut. Breast-feeding is not recommended if the mother has active tuberculosis or chickenpox infections as these can be passed to the baby, as can the AIDS virus. Women taking some antibiotics, TRANQUILLIZERS, hormonal medicine, anti-cancer drugs, radioactive medicines or drinking more than 7 units of ALCOHOL per day should avoid breast-feeding.

During breast-feeding the breasts require special care, with particular attention to washing and drying. Creams and lotions can help prevent soreness and cracked nipples. It is important that the baby is latched on to the breast correctly. It should have the nipple well back in the mouth with the lips around the areola. The mouth is then on the breast tissue instead of the nipple. The baby squeezes the nipple against the palate with its tongue, and this draws milk into its mouth. An infant soon acquires this natural skill. Feeding on demand appears to be the best way of nourishment, and the baby should be allowed to feed from both breasts. Milk can be expressed and kept in the fridge for 48 hours, or can be frozen if required. Breast-feeding may act as a method of CONTRACEPTION as it changes the levels of HORMONES and prevents OVULATION, but it is unreliable, particularly when the baby starts to be weaned. A woman may be ovulating even if menstrual periods are absent. Effectiveness in preventing pregnancy is 60–75 per cent.

Breast-feeding problems generally arise because of excess milk production, sore nipples or an infection. If too much milk is produced, the breasts become engorged. This is eased by feeding or expressing milk by hand or with a pump. Engorged breasts can make it difficult for the baby to latch on properly, and some milk may need to be expressed first. The condition can be eased by bathing the breasts in warm water, applying a hot compress and stroking. Engorgement can occur at any time if the breasts are not emptied of milk, e.g. if the baby misses a feed. As mentioned above, breast-feeding occurs because of the stimulation of nerve endings during suckling, resulting in the let-down reflex. Problems may arise occasionally if the baby is not properly latched on to the breast and so the necessary production of hormones is not triggered. Rarely, a woman may not produce oxytocin at all, and this can be overcome by using a nasal spray containing the hormone. The flow of milk can be affected by the mother's state of mind and will decrease if she is stressed or unhappy. Reassurance and perseverance may be needed.

Many women suffer from sore or cracked nipples when breast-feeding. This may be caused by incorrect latching-on or by allowing the baby to pull on the nipple, especially when it is releasing its hold on the breast. It is best to stop feeding from the affected breast and apply lotion or oil to the nipple, as advised by a doctor or nurse. Sore or cracked nipples heal faster when exposed to air. Cracked nipples can lead to infection, but using a breast shield allows the baby to feed, affording protection while healing occurs. The most common breast infection is MASTITIS, but a BREAST ABSCESS may also form. A blocked milk duct in the nipple is a problem that can result from a bra that is too tight, engorged breasts or from blockage by dried milk. The breast may feel lumpy and tender, with reddened skin. The blockage may be cleared by feeding and massaging the breast above the affected duct, but to lessen the risk of an abscess a doctor's advice should be sought if the condition does not clear.

breast plastic surgery plastic surgery carried out to increase or reduce BREAST size or to restore breast form after a MASTECTOMY. All forms of breast COSMETIC SURGERY are called mammoplasty. Breast reduction may be cosmetic but is more commonly carried out for medical reasons. Large breasts can cause pain in the back or shoulders and be a source of embarrassment. BREAST-FEEDING may not be possible, and the weight can cause problems with breathing and posture. The surgical procedure is complicated, and the aim is to produce smaller breasts with a similar shape. Many surgeons prefer not to operate until after a woman has completed her family and finished breast-feeding.

The operation takes around 3 hours, with excess fat and breast tissue removed and the AREOLA and NIPPLE repositioned. Scars are unavoidable but differ in appearance from one woman to another. There is pain and swelling for up to 6 weeks, and lifting, stretching and sport must be avoided. However, there are fewer complications with breast reduction than with breast enlargement. There may be loss of sensation in the NIPPLES or fat deposits and formation of an ulcer at the site of the scar. Most of these problems resolve with time or treatment. Breast enlargement is the most common cosmetic breast operation. It is not performed on teenage girls whose breasts are still developing. It is commonly carried out after childbirth once the breasts have shrunk in size. The basic procedure is to place a pouch filled with silicone gel or sterile saline either between the breast and the pectoral muscles or under the pectoral muscles. The operation is usually done under a general anaesthetic and takes about an hour. The scars usually fade, but there may be bruising and soreness around the nipples. The patient needs to stay in hospital for a day, have bandages around the breasts for 5 days and wear a good supporting bra day and night for at least 3 weeks. Swelling may be present for up to 6 weeks, and exercise and stretching should be avoided for a month.

There are potential complications, such as blood collecting around the implant, necessitating removal. The implant may need to be removed if an INFECTION occurs, and it can leak. Saline implants may rupture suddenly. The most common problem is capsule formation, in which fibrous tissue forms around the implant so that it cannot move around. This can be intensely painful and can be solved only by cracking the capsule under general ANAESTHESIA. It often recurs, and 6 per cent of women have to have implants removed. There is also a risk of stray silicone leaking from the implant and moving to another part of the body. There are conflicting views as to whether silicone implants increase the risks of BREAST CANCER, cause AUTOIMMUNE DISEASE or reduce detection of cancerous lumps. Many women have MAMMOGRAPHY prior to the operation and follow-up checks to ensure all is well. After breast enlargement, a woman is normally still able to breast-feed. A related operation is a breast lift, where sagging breasts are altered by removing stretched and excess skin. While there is quite a lot of scarring initially, this generally fades and there is little pain but some restriction to initial postoperative activity.

Breast reconstruction is generally carried out after a MASTECTOMY to produce a breast mound that feels natural and is a similar size and shape to the remaining breast. The timing of the reconstruction operation varies, as many doctors like to wait to see if CHEMO-THERAPY or RADIOTHERAPY is necessary. Healing and overall success of reconstruction procedures are affected by these treatments. The type of reconstruction depends on the original mastectomy. If sufficient breast muscle and skin are left, a silicone implant can be used or a similar procedure carried out involving tissue expansion. A silicone bag is inserted under the chest muscle, and it is gradually inflated with saline over an 8-week period. The bag may be replaced with an implant or may be left alone. It results in a similar breast to the original, and women who have had radiotherapy can undergo this procedure. If the mastectomy was more extensive and too little skin is left for an implant, a section of skin and muscle may be taken from the back or abdomen. This is attached at the breast site and used to rebuild the breast with an implant. While this is major surgery with a recovery period of up to three months, it can help to restore a woman's confidence in her body image and bring peace of mind.

breast self-examination the examination by a woman of her own BREASTS in order to know their normal feel and appearance so that she is better able to detect any abnormalities that may warrant investigation. It is best carried out once a month before the menstrual period and self-examination is recommended for all women from age 20. If MENSTRUATION has ceased, breast examination should still be carried out on a monthly basis. Self-examination is done in two ways: inspection and feeling the breasts.

Method of breast self-examination: (1) Look into a mirror, undressed to the waist. Study the breasts and become familiar with their normal appearance. Look at skin texture, height and appearance of the NIPPLES, etc. Check for any unusual differences. (2) Look at each breast for any unusual irregularity in shape, drawing in or retraction of the nipple, dimpling of the skin, changes in skin colour or texture, or VEINS more prominent than normal. This should be done with the arms in different positions: (a) by the side; (b) hands on the waist; (c) arms raised above the head; (d) hands clasped around the head. (3) Squeeze each nipple gently to check for any bleeding or unusual discharge. (4) Checking the breasts by touch is carried out while standing up and/or lying down. It may be done in the bath or shower when the skin is wet. Raise the right arm and use the left hand to explore the right breast in a clockwise motion. With the fingers flat, feel the breast for any unusual lump, knot, mass, thickening, tenderness or other change. Repeat for the other breast. Examine the nipple in a similar manner. (5) Feel in each armpit for any enlarged LYMPH nodes. Hold the left arm by the side and slide the right hand into the armpit and on down the ribs. Repeat on the other side using the left hand with the right arm by the side.

breech birth the most common form of ABNORMAL PRESENTATION. It occurs when the baby's buttocks are the emerging part of its body and happens in approximately 5 per cent of all deliveries. Most breech labours, while presenting some difficulties, result in the birth of a normal baby. There are three main breech positions: full breech, where the buttocks present, the thighs are flexed and the knees bent; back breech, where the thighs are flexed and the legs are upwards; and footing breech, where the thighs are poorly flexed and one or both of the baby's feet present first. Breech babies must be delivered in hospital, and if the condition is recognized in the last few weeks of PREGNANCY, then an attempt may be made to turn the baby by external VERSION, manoeuvring the baby from the outside and turning it head-down. Even if this is successful, the baby often turns back to a breech position. DELIVERY of a breech baby may be more difficult as the largest section, the head, is delivered last so a greater pelvic diameter is needed. If problems arise, FORCEPS may be used to deliver the head, as the baby may try and breathe while still in the BIRTH CANAL. A CAESAREAN SECTION may be necessary in some cases (16 per cent of breech births in the UK but more common in the USA).

bulimia nervosa a condition in which a woman alternately overeats in a binge and then diets to extreme, starves herself, exercises excessively, induces VOMITING or uses laxatives. It generally occurs in women in their twenties, who have low self-esteem and wish to have a thin figure. Women with bulimia know they have a problem but feel too guilty or ashamed to confront it. Like ANOREXIA NERVOSA, bulimia can develop because of the western social pressure to be thin, conflicting messages about food, unhappiness and a need to feel in control. The sufferer generally views herself as fat and starts on an eating binge because of DEPRESSION. The eating is often kept secret, and the person then feels ashamed and disgusted with herself, which triggers the purging. This becomes a vicious circle and leads to VITAMIN and mineral deficiencies, damage to teeth caused by acid erosion, acid stomach, and mouth and gastric ulcers. Also, swollen ankles and fingers, menstrual problems and BREAST tenderness can result. Severe bulimics may suffer kidney damage, muscle weakness and epileptic fits. The binging/purging routine occupies much of a sufferer's time, but most are still able to function well. The incidence of the condition is difficult to determine as sufferers are usually secretive. Treatment may involve self-help groups, PSYCHOTHERAPY, support from partner or family, and possibly ANTIDEPRESSANTS. Over 90 per cent of people with bulimia are women, and diabetic people are more prone to developing it. Recent work has found that 75 per cent of women affected also have POLYCYSTIC OVARIAN SYNDROME, but it is not known if or how these conditions are linked.

bunion an abnormal enlargement of the joint at the base of a big toe, caused by INFLAMMATION of the bursa, the soft tissue pad that limits friction near the joint. There is thickening of the skin, pain, swelling and lateral displacement of the big toe. It is normally caused by wearing ill-fitting, high-heeled shoes and needs treatment by a chiropodist. In severe cases, surgery may be required.

C

Caesarean section (C section, surgical delivery, abdominal delivery) DELIVERY of a baby through an incision in the UTERUS. It has been performed since ancient times and is a major operation. It may be the planned method if the baby is BREECH or lying in a transverse position, or if the mother has certain medical conditions, e.g. DIABETES, active HERPES infection, HYPERTENSION or HEART DISEASE. Also, if the PLACENTA is incorrectly sited, as in PLACENTA PRAEVIA, the baby is too large to travel down the BIRTH CANAL, or there is an infection in the uterus, RHESUS INCOMPATIBILITY, drug addiction or a SEXUALLY TRANSMITTED DISEASE in the mother. An emergency Caesarean may be performed if there are weak uterine CONTRACTIONS, PROLAPSED CORD, foetal distress, PROLONGED LABOUR, ECLAMPSIA or PRE-ECLAMPSIA, ABRUPTIO PLACENTAE or any combination of these factors. A previous Caesarean section may require this method for subsequent babies, but this view is changing, and a 'trial labour', where natural LABOUR is allowed to proceed as long as there are no problems, is becoming more popular. An old belief was that the scar from the first Caesarean would open during labour, but this is unusual with a horizontal incision.

The operation itself requires an EPIDURAL or general anaesthetic, shaving of PUBIC HAIR and a catheter inserted into the BLADDER to drain URINE. An intravenous drip is used to give fluids, and a screen blocks the woman's view of the operation. A horizontal incision is made low down in the uterus, above the CERVIX, and the amniotic fluid is drawn off. The baby is gently lifted out of the uterus, the UMBILICAL CORD is cut and the placenta removed, and the uterine and abdominal walls are stitched up separately. If the baby lies in an unusual position a vertical incision may be used, but this is uncommon. The horizontal cut involves less loss of BLOOD during surgery, less chance of rupture in subsequent pregnancies or vaginal deliveries, easier repair, and reduced risk of postoperative infection. If a woman has been looking forward to a vaginal delivery, a

Caesarean section may disappoint her. It is helpful if her partner
describes the birth in detail, as this helps the mother to accept what
has happened. It helps to prepare for a Caesarean delivery in case
it is needed. A Caesarean affects the baby beneficially in that it
does not have to go through the birth canal and so does not have
the squashed appearance that can result from a vaginal delivery. A
Caesarean baby has a rounded head and smooth facial features
but often needs more time to adjust to the outside world because
of the sudden exit from the uterus. The journey through the birth
canal normally helps to clear amniotic fluid from the baby's lungs
and also stimulates blood circulation.

cancer a term for a range of diseases in which there is uncontrolled
growth of MALIGNANT cells. Certain cells start to proliferate and to
form a tumour that may invade surrounding tissues and spread by
METASTASIS to form secondary growths in other parts of the body.
Cancer develops in phases, starting with initiation then promotion
and progression to form a malignant tumour. Initiation occurs when
DNA molecules inside a cell are attacked by a carcinogen. This
substance can cause irreversible damage to DNA in a very short
time, but some cancers develop without this taking place. The change
in DNA that results is called a mutation. Carcinogens may be natural
or synthetic in origin and include a wide range of substances to
which people are inevitably exposed. Damage to DNA is normally
repaired, but if this does not occur, disease can progress. Initiation
may occur as a result of many minute mutations occuring continually.

In the promotion phase, a cell with a mutation undergoes a
number of chain reactions to produce a cancer cell. The body loses
control of the cell, and it starts to divide and proliferate to form a
tumour composed of genetically identical units. Substances that
promote cell division and proliferation can act as promoters. These
include excessive OESTROGEN, arsenic, epoxides, overexposure to
sunlight and lack of VITAMIN A. The promotion stage is often called
PRECANCEROUS. Progression or clonal evolution follows, in which
the cells in the tumour produce clones of cells. These are slightly
different from the original tumour and from each other. The cells

have a high division rate and may move into other tissues, i.e. metastasize to other areas of the body. When examined under a microscope, the cells look abnormal and disorganized (DYSPLASIA). They are pre-malignant if they have not infiltrated other tissues, but if this has occured, they are termed malignant and cancerous. The promotion and progression phases are difficult, if not impossible, to separate as the process is a continuum.

Cancers exist in many different forms and are classified according to the cells that gave rise to them. The most common types are carcinomas of the skin, GLANDS and the MUCOUS MEMBRANES lining the respiratory, urinary and gastrointestinal systems. Sarcomas develop from connective tissues, cartilage, muscles, and membranes covering muscles and fat, and are less common. Lymphomas are cancers of the lymph nodes while leukaemia affects the white BLOOD cells. The treatment of each type is different, as is the cause and specific progression of the disease. In the UK, the commonest cancers are LUNG CANCER, BREAST CANCER and SKIN CANCER.

In women, cancers of the reproductive system comprise 50 per cent of all cases, but the commonest is lung cancer, caused by smoking, including passive smoking. Research has shown that there may be an inherited predisposition to certain cancers in a woman's genetic make up. Many cancers are curable if detected at an early stage, thus BREAST SELF-EXAMINATION and regular CERVICAL SMEAR TESTS are recommended for women. Further work will increase the effectiveness of screening programmes and treatment of familial cancers. Cancer is treated with surgery, CHEMOTHERAPY, RADIOTHERAPY and HORMONE therapy, and some people use complementary therapies, which can often work well in conjunction with conventional medical treatment. (*See also* CERVICAL CANCER; COLORECTAL CANCER; DYSPLASIA; ENDOMETRIAL CANCER; INFLAMMATORY BREAST CANCER; OVARIAN CANCER; PAGET'S DISEASE OF THE NIPPLE; PELVIC CANCER; PRECANCEROUS; UTERINE CANCER; VAGINAL CANCER; VULVAR CANCER).

cataract a cloudiness that develops in the lens of the eye. They usually affect both eyes and are common in people over 60. The location of the cataract determines the amount of blurring and dimming of vision that occurs. More women develop cataracts because of their greater longevity. Any reduction in vision can be treated with CONTACT LENSES or spectacles, but a cataract can be successfully treated by surgery. The cloudy lens is removed and replaced with a plastic implant, and while care must be taken to avoid direct bright light, vision is greatly improved. People with DIABETES are particularly predisposed to developing cataracts.

cauterization the use of chemicals or heat to destroy cells. It is used to treat GENITAL WARTS, CERVICITIS and PRECANCEROUS LESIONS of the cervix. The process is mildly painful, may cause swelling and leads to a vaginal discharge that can last for several weeks. Similar treatment is carried out using CRYOSURGERY or LASER SURGERY. Cauterization is used in TUBAL LIGATION procedures.

celibacy abstaining from any sexual activity.

cerebral palsy a disorder caused by a permanent, nonprogressive brain defect that is present at birth or occurs shortly afterwards. It often results from lack of oxygen in the brain, caused by a very difficult LABOUR or trauma at birth, prematurity, a severe childhood illness, such as meningitis or poisoning with lead or arsenic. Symptoms range in severity and include lack of balance, involuntary movements, speech problems, irregular gait and facial grimacing. Intelligence may be affected, depending on the site of brain damage. The disorder can be helped by physiotherapy and speech therapy and possibly orthopaedic surgery. Women with cerebral palsy have normal MENSTRUATION and FERTILITY and can sustain a PREGNANCY and birth if the disorder is mild.

cervical cancer abnormal growth of MALIGNANT cells in the CERVIX or neck of the UTERUS. It is the second most common female cancer, and it is successfully curable in the early stages.

The cancer cells may be present in the cervix for 4–10 years before becoming invasive, affecting the deeper tissues and giving rise to symptoms. Even when the cancer is invasive but found only in the cervix, there is an 80 per cent chance of a successful cure. Once it spreads through the pelvis to the VAGINA, UTERUS, BLADDER or RECTUM, it is much more difficult to cure. Regular screening by means of a CERVICAL SMEAR TEST is a very important preventive measure. All women from the age of 20, or from when they become sexually active, should have a smear test every 3 years. Symptoms of cervical cancer include bleeding between menstrual periods or after intercourse and the MENOPAUSE. An offensive vaginal discharge or ulceration of the cervix may also indicate cancer.

Treatment depends on the stage of the cancer. A CONE BIOPSY is taken from the cervix by scalpel or laser, and the tissue is examined under a microscope. Treatment methods include CRYOSURGERY, CAUTERIZATION or LASER SURGERY to remove part of the cervix, and HYSTERECTOMY. Both surgical treatment and RADIOTHERAPY give good results. Around 50 per cent of cervical cancer cases are treated with radiotherapy.

This disease is easily detected but its cause is unknown. Some evidence links the presence of GENITAL WARTS, caused by several kinds of human papilloma VIRUS, and infection with HERPES simplex II virus with the development of cervical cancers. Women at risk include those who had SEXUAL INTERCOURSE from an early age and with many different partners, those with pre-existing SEXUALLY TRANSMITTED DISEASES and some racial groups, including black, Puerto Rican and Mexican women. Smoking increases the risk of developing cervical cancer.

cervical cap a rubber or plastic cup that fits over the CERVIX and prevents SPERM from entering the cervical opening. It is one of the BARRIER METHODS of CONTRACEPTION and requires individual fitting. It stays on the cervix by suction and is used with a SPERMICIDE in a manner similar to a DIAPHRAGM. The cap cannot be used if the woman has an unusually long or short cervix, if there is PELVIC INFLAMMATORY DISEASE, VAGINITIS or CERVICITIS. When used correctly, the cervical cap has a success rate of 85–90 per cent.

cervical erosion *see* CERVICITIS.

cervical eversion a condition in which the normal tissue found on the surface of the CERVIX is replaced by that which is usually situated higher in the cervical canal. Some women are born with this condition, but it can also develop when levels of OESTROGEN in the body are high, i.e. during PUBERTY or PREGNANCY and while taking the combined ORAL CONTRACEPTIVE PILL. The symptoms may include

an increased discharge of CERVICAL MUCUS and possibly the presence of BLOOD. These symptoms require investigation to eliminate
other conditions or INFECTIONS. Treatment may not be necessary,
but it may be advisable to destroy the abnormal tissue by
CRYOSURGERY. (*See also* CERVICITIS).

cervical mucus a clear, colourless, alkaline fluid produced by the
CERVIX to lubricate the exterior of the cervical canal. At the onset
of OVULATION more cervical mucus is produced, and it becomes slippery and thinner in texture and may be noticed as a clear or white
discharge. The mucus also becomes more acidic, which helps SPERM
survive in the VAGINA. Cervical mucus contains proteins and sugars
that sustain sperm, and deficiencies can cause female INFERTILITY.
The mucus may be too thick or too little in quantity so that sperm
cannot move easily. The mucus may also contain ANTIBODIES to the
sperm and so prevent FERTILIZATION by mobilizing an immune response.

cervical polyp a small fleshy, tear-shaped growth that develops high
up in the cervical canal, near the entrance to the UTERUS. POLYPS
develop from the mucous lining of the CERVIX and may occur singly
or in groups. They are almost always BENIGN and may or may not
give rise to symptoms that can include cramping pain or bleeding
after intercourse or between periods. They are easily detected as
they normally protrude into the VAGINA and can be removed using
CAUTERIZATION techniques.

cervical smear test a procedure carried out to detect cancerous and
PRECANCEROUS cell changes in the CERVIX. It is a routine examination that should be carried out every 3 years from becoming sexually active or from age 20. It is also used to diagnose viral INFEC-
TIONS of the urinogenital system and SEXUALLY TRANSMITTED DIS-
EASES. A SPECULUM is inserted into the VAGINA and cervical cells are
removed, using a spatula or swab, and transferred to a glass slide
before being sent for laboratory analysis. The results are normally
available after 6 weeks. The woman should not be menstruating or
have SPERM present in the vagina from recent SEXUAL INTERCOURSE.
Smear test results are classified into 4 or 5 categories, from negative to cancerous cells. A result with mild DYSPLASIA means there is

some infection present and regular smear tests are needed. A positive test indicates there are some cell changes that need further investigation but do not necessarily indicate a cancerous or precancerous condition. A COLPOSCOPY and possibly a BIOPSY may be needed, and if cancerous cells are found, treatment for CERVICAL CANCER begins. The smear screening programme is the best method of detecting cervical cancer presently available. (*See also* CONE BIOPSY.)

cervicitis INFLAMMATION of the CERVIX, which can be caused by chemicals, a foreign body (tampon, IUD string, penis), or an INFECTION including SEXUALLY TRANSMITTED DISEASE such as CHLAMYDIA or GONORRHOEA, or it may be of unknown origin. The condition ranges from mild to severe, with copious vaginal discharge, pelvic and BACK PAIN, and pain during intercourse. There may be slight bleeding after intercourse. A sample of cells is obtained by a CERVICAL SMEAR TEST. Treatment depends on the cause but may include sulphonamide creams and antibiotic pessaries. The woman's partner also requires treatment. If the problem persists, abnormal tissue on the surface of the cervix may be removed by CRYOSURGERY, LASER SURGERY, CONE BIOPSY or CAUTERIZATION. The discharge may block the passage of SPERM up the cervical canal and prevent PREGNANCY. Alternative therapies include VITAMIN E pessaries and the use of spermicidal creams and jellies to soothe inflammation and aid healing.

cervicography a technique used to detect abnormalities of the CERVIX that do not show up in a CERVICAL SMEAR TEST. A photographic image is taken of the cervix by a camera called a cerviscope. The image produced is called a **cervigram**, and it is analysed by experts in COLPOSCOPY. The technique is fairly new and is still being tested but seems to be an effective screening method for CANCER.

cervix the lower section of the UTERUS, which protrudes into the VAGINA. It is known as the neck of the uterus, and the cervical canal passes through it, linking the uterus and the vagina. The cervix is lined with many small GLANDS that produce CERVICAL MUCUS. The consistency of these secretions changes in response to hormonal influences during the MENSTRUAL CYCLE and can provide a method of determining the time of OVULATION (*see* NATURAL FAMILY PLANNING). A CYST may form if one of the glands becomes blocked. The lower end of the cervix has an opening called the external os, and before childbirth it is about 5 mm in diameter. It dilates to 10 cm during LABOUR and never regains its former shape, changing to a slit approximately 7 mm long. Normally the cervix is pink in colour but turns bluish in pregnancy because of an increased BLOOD supply (CHANDWICK'S SIGN). The cervix is liable to several conditions of which CERVICAL CANCER is the most serious. Others include CERVICAL EVERSION, CERVICAL POLYPS, CERVICITIS and DYSPLASIA. (*See also* INCOMPETENT CERVIX).

Chandwick's sign a colour change in the tissues of the CERVIX and vaginal entrance that is used to help diagnose PREGNANCY. These tissues are usually pink but during pregnancy assume a purplish, dusky colour that deepens progressively. The colour changes are most apparent in second and subsequent pregnancies.

chemotherapy treatment of infectious and other diseases with chemical substances or drugs. It is generally applied to drugs used to treat CANCER. Chemotherapeutic drugs are very powerful and kill cancer cells in the original tumour, as well as any stray cells that have broken away from the main growth. Unfortunately, chemotherapy also affects healthy cells. The drugs are most effective against cells that are actively growing, including tumour cells, white BLOOD cells, hair follicles, and several gastrointestinal tissues, especially MUCOUS MEMBRANES. Hence the dosage of these drugs needs to be carefully monitored so that cancerous cells are destroyed while limiting damage to healthy tissue. Cancer drugs work in different ways, with some stopping cell growth and others preventing cell division. Cancer drugs may be used singly or in combination, and each may be more effective against certain forms of the disease. Chemotherapy is administered by mouth or intravenously, each day, week or month, depending on the type of cancer and its stage of progression.

Some cancers require cyclical treatment or continuous infusion by drugs over a period of a few days. All these treatments have SIDE-EFFECTS as the drugs are very toxic. The most common ones are NAUSEA, VOMITING, skin rashes, mouth ulcers and hair loss. Hair loss can be lessened or prevented by keeping the scalp cool during chemotherapy. Altered menstrual periods are possible during chemotherapy, and a reduction in sperm count can occur in males (*see* ARTIFICIAL INSEMINATION). Treatment with such powerful drugs can have serious toxic effects. White blood cell production by the BONE MARROW is reduced, and there are decreased numbers of blood platelets. Fibrosis (death) of liver tissue, CYSTITIS and, over a longer period, the development of ACUTE leukaemia and other cancers may occur. Chemotherapy is used as a primary treatment and to treat a cancer that has, or is thought to have, spread. Also, following removal of a tumour to kill stray cancerous cells and to reduce symptoms and prolong life when the cancer is incurable.

childbearing age the years from first OVULATION following MENARCHE (average age 12½) to the MENOPAUSE (average age 50). The ideal years for childbearing are the late teens and twenties. Women under 16 and over 34 are considered at greater risk when pregnant. There is an increased risk of developing conditions such as ECLAMPSIA or PLACENTA PRAEVIA after 34, and LABOUR and DELIVERY may be more difficult. The chances of abnormality in the baby increase with age, including DOWN'S SYNDROME, cleft palate, SPINA BIFIDA, CEREBRAL PALSY and congenital heart defects.

chlamydia a SEXUALLY TRANSMITTED DISEASE caused by the bacterium, *Chlamydia trachomatis*, the most common in the western world, with about 170,000 new cases in the UK every year alone. *Chlamydia* is a bacterium that resembles a VIRUS in that it is dependent on host cells for growth and reproduction. It lives inside human cells and so cannot be detected by normal diagnostic tests.

Advances in testing have shown just how widespread chlamydia is in the general population. The bacteria may live in the mouth, eyes, liver, lungs and throat but are normally found in adults in the VAGINA, urinary tract and RECTUM. It is a highly infectious organism and easily transferred from person to person. It affects the CERVIX and URETHRA, but in 70 per cent of women there are no outward symptoms. Even if symptoms do develop, such as painful and frequent urination and vaginal discharge, they are easily confused with those of THRUSH, CYSTITIS or HERPES. If untreated, chlamydia

can move up the reproductive system to cause PELVIC INFLAMMA-
TORY DISEASE in which the FALLOPIAN TUBES may be damaged, leading to INFERTILITY. It may also be responsible for ECTOPIC PREGNANCY.
Chlamydia during pregnant can be passed on to the infant during
DELIVERY, causing chlamydial conjunctivitis or pneumonia in the
baby. Chlamydia commonly affects both HETEROSEXUAL and HOMO-
SEXUAL men and may cause infertility. Testing for the disease is quick
and effective. Oral antibiotics for 1–3 weeks clears the infection,
but all sexual partners must be screened and treated to prevent re-
infection. Using barrier contraceptives such as CONDOMS or a DIA-
PHRAGM help. Women with multiple sexual partners and those taking the ORAL CONTRACEPTIVE PILL may be at increased risk of infection although the reasons for the latter are not known.

chloasma a pattern of skin pigmentation that may develop during
PREGNANCY. Brown patches may appear on the bridge of the nose,
cheeks, forehead and neck, and they normally fade and disappear
within 3 months of LABOUR. They are thought to result from increased production of the pigment melatonin because of higher
levels of OESTROGEN and PROGESTERONE (female HORMONES) in the
body. Coloured women may find that they develop patches of paler
skin during pregnancy rather than increased pigmentation.

cholesterol a fatty insoluble molecule (sterol) that is widely found in
the body and is synthesized from saturated fatty acids in the liver.
Cholesterol is an important substance in the body, being a compo-
nent of cell membranes and a precursor in the production of steroid HORMONES (sex hormones) and bile salts. An elevated level of
BLOOD cholesterol is associated with ARTERIOSCLEROSIS, which may
result in high BLOOD PRESSURE and coronary thrombosis, and this
may occur with DIABETES. There appears to be a relationship between the high consumption of saturated animal fats (which contain cholesterol) in the western diet and the greater incidence of
coronary HEART DISEASE among, for example, Western Europeans
and North Americans. It is generally recommended that people in
these countries should reduce their consumption of saturated fat
and look for alternatives in the form of unsaturated fats, which are
found in vegetable oils. In the blood, cholesterol forms complexes

with proteins to produce lipoproteins. There are two main forms of cholesterol lipoprotein—high-density lipoprotein (HDL) and low-density lipoprotein (LDL). LDL is the form that promotes the build-up of fatty plaques in ARTERY walls, leading to higher risk of arteriosclerosis, heart disease and STROKE.

chorion the outermost membrane round a fertilized EGG, which develops finger-like projections called villi about 2 weeks after CONCEPTION. The villi develop into the PLACENTA, which embeds itself into the uterine lining and allows exchange of nutrients and waste products between the maternal and foetal BLOOD supply.

chorion biopsy an alternative name for CHORIONIC VILLUS SAMPLING.

chorionic villus sampling (CVS) a special prenatal test used to detect genetic abnormalities in the FOETUS. It is carried out between 10 and 12 weeks of PREGNANCY, earlier than AMNIOCENTESIS.

There are two ways of testing. In one, a catheter is inserted into the outside edge of the PLACENTA via the cervical canal and CERVIX. A sample of chorionic tissue is removed and the cells examined. Cells of the chorionic villi have the same GENETIC CODE as the foetus, so examining them can reveal if the EMBRYO has a genetic defect. In the second, a sample of chorionic tissue is obtained by inserting a needle through the abdominal wall and into the placenta. Instead of removing amniotic fluid, as in the amniocentesis test, chorionic tissue is removed. Both techniques are carried out guided by ULTRASOUND. The tissue does not need to be cultured and so results of the test are available in 24 to 48 hours. As the tests are carried out earlier in pregnancy, an ABORTION can be offered if it is considered advisable.

CVS carries a higher risk of MISCARRIAGE (2.5 per cent) than amniocentesis and is normally offered to women at risk of having a DOWN'S SYNDROME baby or one with SICKLE-CELL ANAEMIA, THALASSAEMIA, CYSTIC FIBROSIS, HAEMOPHILIA or MUSCULAR DYSTROPHY. Huntington's chorea and congenital metabolic defects can also be detected by CVS testing.

chromosomes the rod-like structures present in the nucleus of every body cell that carry the genetic information or GENES. Each human body cell contains 23 pairs of CHROMOSOMES (apart from the SPERM and OVUM), half derived from the mother and half from the father. Each chromosome consists of a coiled double filament (double helix) of DNA, with genes carrying the genetic information arranged linearly along its length. The genes determine all the characteristics of each individual. Of the pairs of chromosomes, 22 are the same in males and females. The 23rd pair are the sex chromosomes, and males have 1 X-CHROMOSOME and one Y-CHROMOSOME whereas females have 2 X-CHROMOSOMES. Genetic replication is subject to possible mistakes, leading to chromosome defects. Three-quarters of these defects are normally considered undesirable, and some MIS-CARRIAGES are thought to be caused by chromosome abnormalities. (*See also* BIRTH DEFECTS; CHROMOSOME TESTING; GENETIC CODE; GENETIC SCREENING).

chromosome testing tests carried out to determine if a person carries an abnormal GENE for a certain disease or to discover the genetic make-up of a FOETUS and detect any abnormalities. Tests for HAEMOPHILIA, SICKLE-CELL ANAEMIA, CYSTIC FIBROSIS or DOWN'S SYNDROME can be carried out in prospective parents if there is a family history of one of these genetic disorders. This can be done by taking a BLOOD sample or a cell swab from the buccal (mouth) cavity and culturing the cells. IN VITRO FERTILIZATION and screening of fertilized eggs can help some high-risk couples to have a normal child. Babies can be tested for many disorders while still in the UTERUS. (*See also* BIRTH DEFECTS; AMNIOCENTESIS; CHORIONIC VILLUS SAMPLING; UMBILICAL CORD SAMPLING.)

chronic an illness, INFECTION or INFLAMMATION that persists for a long period of time (*compare* ACUTE).

chronic pain intractable pain that lasts for 6 months or more and does not respond well to any conventional treatment. It can result from surgery, serious injury or diseases such as ENDOMETRIOSIS, PELVIC INFLAMMATORY DISEASE or ARTHRITIS. It can severely curtail the sufferer's life and may lead to drug dependency or the long-term use of ANALGESICS. The pain may be eased by physiotherapy or some alternative medical techniques such as ACUPUNCTURE, hypnosis and counselling. CHRONIC pain requires different treatment from ACUTE pain and skill in its long-term management.

circumcision the surgical removal of the foreskin of the penis in males and the CLITORIS or the hood of the clitoris in females. Female circumcision is still carried out on young girls for cultural or religious reasons in many Islamic countries in Africa, although it is usually illegal and never medically justified.

clitoris a small cylindrical structure near the pubic BONE, which is enclosed in a hood composed of the LABIA minora. It is the female equivalent of the male penis and contains many nerve endings and erectile tissue that stiffens with increased blood flow during SEXUAL AROUSAL. The clitoris is very sensitive and becomes engorged with blood during sexual stimulation, increasing in size, but even then it is usually less than 2.5 cm long. The clitoris is the primary focus of ORGASM in a woman, and its only known function is for sexual pleasure. Since the 19th century, operations to remove the clitoris and/or surrounding tissue were carried out to cure 'female hysteria' and to stop MASTURBATION, but today such surgery is regarded as totally unnecessary and cruel. Rarely, the clitoris needs to be removed in cases of CANCER where the external genitals are affected. (*See also* CIRCUMCISION; VULVAR CANCER.)

coitus an alternative name for SEXUAL INTERCOURSE.

coitus interruptus (interrupted intercourse) a method of CONTRACEPTION where the man removes his penis from the woman's VAGINA before he ejaculates. It is an unreliable method of contraception (approximately 75 per cent effective) and may lead to sexual ANXIETY in one or both partners.

cold sore a tiny blister that is usually found on the lips or nostrils but may occur on the cheeks or around the eye. Cold sores are caused by the HERPES simplex I VIRUS, which is transferred from person to person by kissing or skin contact. The virus lives in the nerve endings in the skin and becomes active only when there is a rise in skin temperature caused by a FEVER, sunlight or an INFECTION such as a cold. The skin starts to tingle and becomes tender, then a small blister appears, and within 24 hours it grows larger, bursts and forms a crust. The blister takes 10 to 14 days to heal, and it may leave a scar. Treatment is a matter of personal choice but no action can reduce the time taken for the sore to heal. If a cold sore is near the eye, it is more dangerous as ulcers can form on the front of the eyeball. Special treatment is needed to stop any damage occurring.

colorectal cancer a growth of MALIGNANT cells in the large intestine, colon and RECTUM. It is becoming increasingly common and has a high fatality rate. This is largely because the early symptoms are not particularly prominent and because bowel disorders cause embarrassment, preventing people from seeking early treatment. Colorectal CANCER has very few early warning signs, but these include dark brown or tarry stools, flecks of BLOOD in stools, changes in bowel habits, tiredness, lethargy, abdominal pain and indigestion. A doctor may first carry out a rectal examination and then refer the patient to a specialist. Diagnostic tests include a barium enema and X-RAY, which show any irregularities in the intestine, or colonoscopy/sigmoidoscopy, which uses fibre-optic tubes to view the large intestine.

If cancer is found in most cases it is treated surgically. Colorectal cancers are slow to spread, and recovery is good if detected early. CHEMOTHERAPY and RADIOTHERAPY are used if it has spread. A COLOSTOMY may be necessary with some types of surgery. Women over 60 with a family history of intestinal POLYPS or pre-existing intestinal disease (such as ulcerative colitis) are at greater risk. A low-fibre, high-fat diet is believed to increase the risk. The best means of prevention is attention to diet, and high-fibre, low-fat foods are recommended. After the age of 50, an annual rectal examination may help.

colostomy a surgical opening of the large intestine (colon) through the abdominal wall so solid waste (faeces) can be discharged. This operation is performed when the colon or RECTUM is diseased or injured and cannot be treated medically. Diseases such as COLORECTAL CANCER, ulcerative colitis, Crohn's disease and diverticulitis often require colostomy. BIRTH DEFECTS are another reason why this operation may be necessary.

colposcopy a technique for examining the CERVIX and VAGINA. This procedure is normally carried out after an abnormal CERVICAL SMEAR TEST and allows a magnified view of the surface of the cervix. A doctor views the cell type, pattern of blood vessels and white patches on the cervix to help determine PRECANCEROUS or cancerous changes.

This technique can identify an area of abnormal cells, and a sample can then be taken for investigation. The results of a colposcopy help determine further treatment, such as a CONE BIOPSY, or it may show CERVICAL EVERSION as the cause of the abnormal cells. The colposcopy procedure takes 15 to 20 minutes and is painless. (*See also* CERVICAL CANCER).

conception the FERTILIZATION of an EGG or OVUM by a SPERM in the FALLOPIAN TUBE. The fertilized egg is called a ZYGOTE.

condom or **sheath** a BARRIER METHOD of contraception consisting of a thin rubber sheath that covers the penis during SEXUAL INTERCOURSE and traps ejaculated SPERM. It is one of the oldest types of contraceptive. Condoms help to reduce the spread of SEXUALLY TRANSMITTED DISEASE such as GONORRHOEA, HERPES, SYPHILIS, CHLAMYDIA and AIDS. They are readily available and can be obtained free from family planning clinics and some GPs' surgeries and are around 95–98 per cent effective in preventing PREGNANCY. They should display the BSI kitemark on the packet as this ensures that they have been tested to a high standard. A type of condom that can be used by women has become available recently. It is a soft polyurethane sheath that lines the vagina and extends over the LABIA. It is inserted before sex and provides excellent protection against sexually transmitted diseases. At the moment there is no available data for its effectiveness.

cone biopsy (conization) a method used to remove a cone-shaped piece of tissue from the CERVIX for investigation and examination under a microscope. This surgical technique is carried out if one or more CERVICAL SMEAR TESTS indicate DYSPLASIA or the presence of PRECANCEROUS or cancerous cells in the cervix. A cone biopsy is done if a COLPOSCOPY has not isolated the abnormal cells. The surgery is performed under a general anaesthetic, and a D AND C may be carried out at the same time to check the lining of the UTERUS for the presence of CANCER. The edges of the cervix are stitched with stitches that are readily absorbed during healing. A cone biopsy may remove the entire cancerous area, but further surgery and/or RADIOTHERAPY may be required. The patient undergoing this procedure will experience some BLOOD loss, and other problems can arise.

A cone biopsy narrows the cervical canal and may reduce FERTIL-
ITY. There can be inadequate production of CERVICAL MUCUS, problems delivering a baby, or the MENSTRUAL FLOW may be impeded.
The surgery may lead to cervical incompetence, which can give rise
to MISCARRIAGE in future pregnancies. These potential problems
mean that colposcopy is used in preference if at all possible. (*See
also* CERVICAL CANCER; INCOMPETENT CERVIX.)

congenital defect a defect or condition that is present in a baby at
birth. (*See also* BIRTH DEFECTS.)

congenital infection an INFECTION that is present in a baby at birth.
It is normally acquired from the mother before or during DELIVERY.
Various bacteria or VIRUSES can be transmitted to the FOETUS across
the PLACENTA, including those that cause GERMAN MEASLES and
chicken pox, or to the baby as it passes through the BIRTH CANAL.
Some SEXUALLY TRANSMITTED DISEASES such as CHLAMYDIA, GENITAL
HERPES, GONORRHOEA and AIDS can be transmitted to the baby as it
passes down the birth canal if the mother is infected. A baby can
also be born with drug or ALCOHOL addiction if its mother has abused
these. (*See also* BIRTH DEFECTS; DRUG USE.)

constipation hard, infrequent stools that are difficult and painful
to eliminate. Most cases of constipation are caused by the wrong
diet, with too little fibre, insufficient fluid intake and lack of EX-
ERCISE. CHRONIC constipation, in which a person may be dependent on laxatives, may indicate a disease or disorder, including DIA-
BETES, an intestinal obstruction, HAEMORRHOIDS, anal fissure and
gastrointestinal disorders. Constipation can be a problem in PREG-
NANCY because of relaxed bowel muscles and pressure on the colon from the enlarged UTERUS. All types of constipation can be
helped by regular exercise, plenty of fluids and a diet rich in fibre
from fresh fruit, raw vegetables, nuts and wholegrains. Constipation can be caused by medicines such as antacids, diuretic and
some heart drugs, codeine and ORAL CONTRACEPTIVE PILLS. The use
of natural laxatives such as figs or prunes does not usually cause
harm, but it is inadvisable to use laxative drugs for any length of
time. These should always be taken under medical advice. In some
cases an enema may be needed to clear the bowel.

contact dermatitis INFLAMMATION of the skin that results from contact with an irritating agent or substance. Many people are sensitive to the metals in jewellery, particularly nickel, and may develop this condition. Treatment is by means of various creams that may contain steroids.

contact lenses small circles of plastic or glass that are worn on the eyeball and correct problems with vision. They may be 'hard' or 'soft', depending on their composition. Hard lenses allow oxygen to pass through to the cornea but can be worn only for restricted periods, normally around 12 hours. Soft lenses are more than 70 per cent water, so they must be kept wet and can be worn for long periods. No contact lens should be left in place overnight. The main problems that can develop are corneal OEDEMA (swelling of the cornea) caused by lack of oxygen and intolerance of the lens.

contraception literally, 'against CONCEPTION', but some methods prevent FERTILIZATION while others prevent IMPLANTATION and PREGNANCY. (*See also* BARRIER METHOD; BREAST-FEEDING; COITUS INTERRUPTUS; INTRAUTERINE DEVICE; NATURAL FAMILY PLANNING; ORAL CONTRACEPTIVE PILL; SPERMICIDE; STERILIZATION.)

contraction the rhythmic tightening of muscles normally used to describe those of the of the UTERUS during LABOUR. Contractions happen involuntarily and act to push the baby down through the BIRTH CANAL. Small, trial contractions, called BRAXTON-HICK CONTRACTIONS, occur in PREGNANCY from around the 34th week. In labour, the contractions are regular in duration and rhythm. In the first stage, short contractions may be separated by 10–20 minute periods and may feel like discomfort in the back and lower abdomen. They gradually increase in strength and duration, with a shorter time between each one. By the end of the first stage of labour, they may last 1–1½ minutes and be only 30 seconds apart. After full cervical dilation the contractions may last 50–100 seconds and recur every 2–3 minutes. The contractions stop for a few minutes after DELIVERY of the baby and then resume to expel the PLACENTA from the uterus. Abdominal massage helps the placenta with this, and the contractions felt at this time are sometimes called AFTERPAINS. These may continue for several days and can require mild pain relief and occur while the uterus is regaining its normal size. They are also stimulated by OXYTOCIN, the HORMONE produced during BREAST-FEEDING. Uterine contractions in labour still occur in women having a regional anaesthetic and in paraplegics with no muscle control in the pelvis. Weaker uterine contractions may be felt as menstrual CRAMPS in non-pregnant women and occur during female ORGASM.

contraindication any factor in the condition of a person that makes a particular treatment or procedure unwise. For example, a woman with a history of HEART DISEASE should not take ORAL CONTRACEPTIVE PILLS.

corpus luteum the structure formed from a ruptured GRAAFIAN FOLLICLE after OVULATION has taken place. The corpus luteum secretes PROGESTERONE (a female HORMONE), which prepares the UTERUS for the IMPLANTATION of a fertilized egg. If this does not occur, the corpus luteum becomes inactive and gradually shrinks into a tiny speck of scar tissue. If an embryo implants and PREGNANCY is established, the corpus luteum is maintained by HUMAN CHORIONIC GONADOTROPHIN, a hormone produced by the PLACENTA. The corpus luteum continues to produce progesterone until around 16 weeks of pregnancy when the placenta takes over this role. The function of the luteum declines and it then disintegrates.

cosmetic surgery the reconstruction of cutaneous or underlying tissues that is performed to remove evidence of ageing, a scar or birthmark, blemish or wrinkle. It is mainly done on the face, neck, nose (rhinoplasty), brow, chin, cheeks or eyelids (blepharoplasty). Body surgery can include abdominoplasty, with removal of fat and skin from the abdomen, or be performed on upper arms, thighs, hips and buttocks. A total body lift and liposuction is where fat is removed from areas of the body. All operations involve general ANAESTHESIA, a degree of hospitalization, discomfort, pain and scarring. For best results, a competent surgeon who is realistic about possible problems and the outcome of surgery is essential. In some cases, attitude to ageing should be changed instead of surgery. (*See also* BREAST PLASTIC SURGERY.)

crab lice *see* PUBIC LICE.

cramp a prolonged and painful spasmodic muscular contraction that occurs in limbs but can also affect internal organs. Leg cramp is common in PREGNANCY, often at night, and during childbirth. Cramp during sleep is common in the elderly and diabetics. Continual repetitive use of certain muscles can result in cramp, e.g. writer's cramp. Menstrual cramps are mild uterine CONTRACTIONS and may arise because of hormonal factors. They may be eased by taking painkillers or supplements of gamma-linolenic acid, which acts against the PROSTAGLANDINS causing the problem.

critical weight the proportion of body fat to lean tissue that seems to be required before MENARCHE commences and regular menstrual periods are maintained. Through ADOLESCENCE, the ratio of lean to fat tissue changes from 5:1 through to 3:1 at menarche. This represents an increase in fat tissue of 125 per cent over 2–3 years. This explains why plump girls usually menstruate at an earlier age than thin ones. The way in which the higher proportion of fat tissue stimulates production of HORMONES is not known, but women with reduced levels of body fat because of ANOREXIA NERVOSA or high levels of physical activity, e.g. athletes or dancers, often have very IRREGULAR PERIODS or none at all (AMENORRHOEA). The MENSTRUAL CYCLE normally resumes if they gain weight.

cryosurgery a technique using extreme cold in a localized part of the body to freeze and destroy unwanted tissue. It is commonly used to treat GENITAL WARTS, some PRECANCEROUS LESIONS of the CERVIX (DYSPLASIA) and some cases of CERVICITIS. It is also used to remove CATARACTS and destroy certain BONE tumours. Cryosurgery is preferred to CAUTERIZATION because it produces a more even level of tissue destruction and causes less scarring, pain and narrowing of the cervical canal.

curettage the removal of thin strands of tissue from the UTERUS or other organ, using an instrument called a curette. (*See also* D AND C; DILATATION AND EVACUATION; VACUUM ASPIRATION.)

Cushing's syndrome a disorder mainly affecting women of CHILD-BEARING AGE and caused by overproduction of the HORMONE cortisol. Symptoms include OBESITY of the face, neck and trunk that develops rapidly, a moon face, excess body hair (HIRSUTISM), ACNE,

STRETCH MARKS of the skin (STRIAE), OLIGOMENORRHOEA or AMEN-
ORRHOEA, a tendency to bruise easily and HYPERTENSION. The disorder can result from malfunctioning of the pituitary or ADRENAL
GLANDS but is usually caused by a PITUITARY GLAND tumour. Treatment includes surgery to remove a tumour, RADIOTHERAPY and removal of one or both adrenal glands. Cortisone replacement therapy
may be required for the rest of the person's life.

cyst an abnormal sac that is filled with fluid or semi-solid matter.
Different varieties of cyst occur, e.g. in the skin, BREASTS, ovaries
and CERVIX. (*See also* BREAST CYST; MASTITIS; OVARIAN CYST; POLY-
CYSTIC OVARIAN SYNDROME.)

cystic fibrosis (CF) an inherited genetic disease in which there is a
disorder of the mucus-secreting GLANDS in the lungs, PANCREAS,
mouth, sweat glands of the skin, and those in the gastrointestinal
tract. The main symptoms are respiratory problems and a failure
to grow despite normal appetite and vigour. Repeated, often severe, respiratory INFECTIONS are common. Treatment is by regular
daily physiotherapy and postural drainage, pancreatic enzyme tablets to make up for inadequate functioning of the pancreas, VITA-
MIN supplements and a high calorie diet to encourage weight gain.
Treatment of secondary infections with antibiotics is very important. Tests for the presence of the GENE that causes the disease can
be done using samples of BLOOD or cells scraped from the mouth
lining. GENETIC SCREENING can be carried out for prospective parents with a family history of the disease. If both carry a defective
gene for CF, there is a 1 in 4 chance of their child being affected.
Survival and treatment of sufferers is improving, but only a few
people with CF survive into their forties. Since the gene and its
CHROMOSOME site were found in the 1980s, research has continued
and gene therapy is now being investigated as a way of curing the
disease. In this a normal gene is inserted into the cells of the lungs,
replacing the defective one so that respiratory and digestive problems gradually diminish. CF is the most common serious genetic
disease in white children with an incidence of 1 in 2000 births. (*See
also* BIRTH DEFECTS; GENETIC COUNSELLING).

cystitis INFLAMMATION of the BLADDER, which may be caused by

bacterial INFECTION or mechanical irritation, a very common ailment contracted by nearly all women at some point in life. The
main symptoms are an urgent need to pass URINE frequently but
with little being passed, a burning or stinging sensation on passing
urine that contains blood, and a dragging pain or pressure in the
lower abdomen. It is frequently caused by infection with the *Escherichia coli*, bacteria that normally live harmlessly in the RECTUM
and are found on skin around the anus. The bacteria can easily
gain access from the rectum to the VAGINA and the urinary tract.
Cystitis is a particular problem in women as the URETHRA is much
shorter than it is in men. It can be caused by SEXUAL INTERCOURSE,
as some positions can irritate the floor of the urethra and bladder.
The use of a DIAPHRAGM can irritate the urethra, as can bubble baths
and chemicals added to some swimming pools. A CYSTOCELE can
contribute to infection as it prevents complete emptying of the bladder and creates an environment in which the bacteria can grow.

Cystitis is common during PREGNANCY as the urethra relaxes under the influence of PROGESTERONE and infections can ascend more
easily. The wearing of nylon tights or tight jeans can cause cystitis
because of pressure or bruising of the urethra. Treatment involves
drinking plenty of water (at least 8 glasses a day) and taking antibiotics. It also helps to make the urine alkaline as the bacteria prefer acid conditions. This is done by adding a teaspoon of baking
soda or bicarbonate of soda to drinking water. A hot water bottle
and painkillers such as paracetamol can help to reduce pain. Cystitis can recur or even become CHRONIC, so adequate fluid intake is
essential to prevent this. Passing urine before and after sexual intercourse can flush out any bacteria introduced into the bladder or
urethra and help in prevention. Correct wiping of the GENITALS from
front to back after urination helps to prevent cystitis. (*See also* DYSU-
RIA).

cystocele (dropped or fallen BLADDER) a PROLAPSE at the base of the
bladder in women. It results in the bulging of the bladder into the
vaginal canal. It generally arises because of weakness of the PELVIC
FLOOR MUSCLES that normally hold the bladder in place, and this
can occur as a result of childbirth. The main symptom of weak-

ened muscles is leaking of URINE, particularly when coughing, sneezing or laughing. A cystocele often leads to repeated urinary infections with symptoms similar to those of CYSTITIS. It is easily diagnosed by PELVIC EXAMINATION, and severe cystocele may be treated effectively with surgery. Minor cases can be improved by doing KEGEL EXERCISES to strengthen the pelvic floor muscles. (*See also* STRESS INCONTINENCE; RECTOCELE; URETHROCELE.

cytotoxic a substance that damages or destroys cells. Cytotoxic drugs are used in the treatment of various forms of CANCER and act by inhibiting cell division. However, they also damage normal cells and hence their use has to be carefully regulated in each individual patient. Cytotoxic drugs may be used in combination with RADIOTHERAPY or on their own.

D

D and C the abbreviation for dilatation and CURETTAGE, one of the most common surgical procedures in women. In a D and C, the CERVIX is dilated using a narrow metal rod and the lining of the UTERUS (ENDOMETRIUM) is scraped off with a curette. Suction may occasionally be used to remove the tissue. A D and C is a method of diagnosing abnormal bleeding, to determine if OVULATION has occurred in cases of INFERTILITY or to detect CANCER of the uterus or FALLOPIAN TUBES. It may be used as a method of ABORTION or to remove uterine ADHESIONS, endometrial polyps and retained placental tissue after childbirth, MISCARRIAGE or abortion. It is helpful in lessening heavy menstrual periods. This procedure is also routine after a STERILIZATION operation and is used to diagnose FIBROIDS. The operation is usually done under general ANAESTHESIA and takes around 20 minutes. After a D and C, a woman may have bleeding for about 14 days and mild cramping pain for a couple of days. Women are advised to avoid vaginal intercourse, the use of tampons and DOUCHING for two weeks, to give the cervix time to get back to its normal closed position. These activities are all a potential source of INFECTION in the cervix or uterus, which is the main complication following this procedure. Any heavy bleeding, abdominal pain, FEVER or foul-smelling vaginal discharge indicates infection and should be treated. Two weeks after a D and C there is usually a postoperative check-up. Other rare complications are perforation of the uterus by a surgical instrument. A D and C is not performed if there is any infection of the uterus, cervix or Fallopian tubes. In some rare cases a D and C can result in the formation of scar tissue in the walls of the uterus. (*See also* DILATATION AND EVACUATION; INCOMPLETE MISCARRIAGE; POLYP; ENDOMETRIOSIS; UTERINE CANCER; UTERINE POLYP; FIBROIDS.)

dandruff a common condition in which the scalp is covered with small flakes of dead skin. The flakes result from an increase in the normal loss of cells from the outermost skin layer. Dandruff is often confused with a type of ECZEMA, seborrhoeic dermatitis, where the scalp is red and inflamed and may weep fluid. Dandruff can normally be cleared by using a medicated shampoo containing tar, sulphur or salicylic acid but, if severe, may need a preparation with zinc pyrithione or selenium sulphide. Frequent washing may resolve some cases. Dandruff can occur caused by under- or overproduction of sebum or oil, changing hormonal levels, or poor blood supply to the scalp.

decompression bubble a device that is fitted round a woman's abdomen during childbirth. It reduces the atmospheric pressure to make the uterine CONTRACTIONS more effective in expelling the baby. A suction pump removes air from the bubble, resulting in the woman's abdomen lifting up and away from her UTERUS so the muscles can work more efficiently. The pump is controlled by the woman, who can switch it on whenever a contraction starts. The decompression bubble is said to make LABOUR more comfortable and speed up DELIVERY. This device is used widely in South Africa and also in some American hospitals.

deep-vein thrombosis a disorder in which a BLOOD CLOT or THROMBUS forms in one of the deep VEINS in the body. In women it generally affects the legs but can arise in the abdomen. The blood clot blocks the vein and causes swelling of the foot, ankle, and lower leg, pain, tenderness and warmth and discoloration of overlying skin. A thrombus is potentially life-threatening as part of the clot (called an embolus) can break away and travel in the BLOOD circulation. If the embolus reaches the lungs it causes a pulmonary EMBO- LISM in which an ARTERY is partially or completely blocked. In the case of partial blockage the amount of blood flowing from the lungs to the heart is reduced and there may be death of lung tissue. A large pulmonary embolism is usually immediately fatal. Antico- agulant drugs are used to treat minor cases, streptokinase may be used to dissolve the clot, or emergency surgery may be necessary. Hence, treatment of a deep-vein thrombosis is designed to deal with the clot before it has time to fragment. Anti-coagulant drugs, which 'thin' the blood and reduce clotting, are given and ANALGESICS for pain. Swelling can be reduced by raising the affected leg, wearing support stockings and by walking about. Weight loss (if overweight) improves the blood circulation, and oral contraceptives must be avoided. A severe deep-vein thrombosis can permanently affect drainage of blood through the veins, and VARICOSE VEINS or a vari- cose ulcer may later develop.

The disorder is fairly uncommon, and women are most at risk following childbirth or major surgery requiring enforced bed rest. There is a tendency for blood to collect in the legs under these cir- cumstances, but to lessen the risk of thrombosis, patients are en- couraged to become mobile as soon as possible or are given physi- otherapy. Women who are overweight, who smoke, who are over 35 or who take combined oral contraceptives (for over 5 years) or hor- mone therapy are at greater risk of deep-vein thrombosis.

delivery the actual birth of a baby, the end result of LABOUR or par- turition.

demand feeding a schedule of BREAST-FEEDING based on the baby's wish to nurse rather than on specific times, e.g. every 3–4 hours. This means frequent feeding, and mothers who breast-feed on de- mand produce more milk than those feeding their babies in a set routine. Demand-fed babies receive more milk per feed and gain more weight than those fed at fixed intervals.

dental problems teeth should be cared for by regular brushing with a good toothbrush and a fluoride toothpaste and by regular flossing. Problems can arise because of GUM DISEASE and the build-up of plaque. Bad breath or halitosis can develop because of food eaten, diseases of the teeth or infections of the lungs, nose and throat. Tooth decay is one of the most common problems and occurs when the tooth enamel breaks down and exposes the layers below. Affected teeth can be treated to remove decay, usually by means of fillings, but may need to be extracted. An ABSCESS can develop round the root of the tooth and is usually painful. Drainage of the abscess and root-canal therapy normally solves the problem and saves the tooth. Grinding of the teeth, particularly at night, is often because of underlying ANXIETY and produces wear and tear. Most dental problems are prevented by good oral HYGIENE, especially daily brushing and regular dental check-ups.

depression an emotional and mental state of extreme sadness, disappointment and frustration that disturbs normal patterns of behaviour. It has a range of severity and is a very common disorder that affects more women than men. Doctors generally distinguish between two types. Reactive depression (also called exogenous) starts as a natural reaction to a stressful situation or event. Reasons include death of a family member, isolation because of unemployment, a marriage problem or financial worries. Endogenous depression, with no obvious cause, can be caused by changing HORMONE levels or can develop after an illness, such as glandular fever or infectious HEPATITIS.

Anyone may feel depressed at some time in life, but depression becomes an illness only when the symptoms are long-lasting or severe enough to interfere with normal functioning over a period of months or years. Symptoms of depression include weepiness, inability to feel pleasure, forgetfulness, low self-esteem, changes in appetite, WEIGHT GAIN or loss, sleep disturbances and INSOMNIA, and HEADACHES. Also, indigestion, restlessness, loss of interest in work, lethargy, feelings of helplessness or hopelessness, ANXIETY, mood shifts, FATIGUE, stooped posture, sad facial expression and inability to think or concentrate. Thoughts of death and suicide can occur in the severely depressed. Treatment depends on the set of symptoms and on the individual involved. Depression can be helped by some ANTIDEPRESSANT drugs, which are particularly beneficial in severe cases but should be taken only for a short period under medical supervision. Hormone therapy, sleeping pills, PSYCHO-THERAPY and electroconvulsive therapy may also be used. Many people believe that depression in some women results from unrealistically high expectations of combining a successful career with family life. Married women often have worse mental health and higher rates of depressive illness than single women and married men. (*See also* POSTNATAL DEPRESSION).

DES (diethylstilbestrol) an artificial OESTROGEN first produced in 1938 and used until 1971 to prevent MISCARRIAGE in early PREGNANCY. This synthetic HORMONE was given to women who had already suffered a previous early miscarriage and has given rise to subsequent problems both in the women and their offspring. Mothers who took this drug appear to have a higher incidence of PELVIC and BREAST CANCER. Daughters born to DES mothers have a 90 per cent chance of having ADENOSIS, an abnormal growth of glandular tissue in the CERVIX and VAGINA. They have a 75 per cent chance of abnormalities of the UTERUS and a higher incidence of clear-cell adenocarcinoma, a rare form of VAGINAL CANCER. In their own pregnancies DES daughters also have an increased risk of an INCOMPETENT CERVIX during pregnancy, which can lead to miscarriage, and they have greater rates of PREMATURE BIRTH.

DES sons have a higher incidence of GENITAL and urinary abnormalities, including CYSTS, undescended testes, underdeveloped testes, low SPERM count, urinary problems and absence of SPERM leading to INFERTILITY. DES sons are advised to see a specialist after PUBERTY and have annual examinations from then on. Mothers who took DES are recommended to examine their BREASTS each month and have yearly breast and PELVIC EXAMINATIONS. DES daughters should undergo pelvic examinations every year after their first menstrual period and have a check-up if they have any unusual bleeding or discharge. A CERVICAL SMEAR TEST, COLPOSCOPY of the vagina and cervix and a SCHILLER TEST should be performed annually. These checks ensure early detection of any problems. DES is currently used in HORMONE REPLACEMENT THERAPY, in the morning-after pill and as treatment for breast and prostate cancer. It is no longer used during pregnancy. (*See also* BREAST SELF-EXAMINATION.)

diabetes (sugar diabetes, diabetes mellitus) a complex metabolic disorder in which the PANCREAS fails to produce enough effective insulin. Insulin is a HORMONE that removes sugar from the BLOOD, enabling it to be stored in the liver and muscles. Without this process, glucose levels in the blood rise alarmingly and body cells lack energy. Cells use fats and proteins as an energy source, and this produces toxic waste products called ketones. If treatment is not administered, cardiac and kidney functioning is affected, leading to a hyperglycaemic coma and possibly death. Symptoms of diabetes include profound thirst, excessive urination, glucose in the URINE, itchiness of the VULVA, soreness and INFLAMMATION of the genital area in women (because of glucose in urine) and loss of weight. Increased hunger, FATIGUE and breath smelling of pear drops (ketones) are further signs of the disorder. Diabetes cannot be cured but it can be controlled either by diet alone, oral medication or by administering insulin. Uncontrolled diabetes can be extremely dangerous, resulting in circulatory problems that can rarely lead to gangrene and loss of limbs, eye problems and possible blindness.

There are at least two forms of diabetes. Type I diabetes (also called insulin-dependent, juvenile-onset) tends to appear in childhood and is caused by an absence of insulin production from the pancreas. This usually requires life-long insulin therapy, and there is a higher risk of developing serious complications. Type II diabetes (also called non-insulin-dependent, maturity-onset) normally affects people after the age of 30 and is slightly more common in women than men. It usually develops gradually, and the body produces insulin but not enough to cope with the levels of carbohydrate and sugar in the diet. The person becomes relatively deficient in insulin and may not suspect diabetes as the condition develops slowly. Levels of sugar and carbohydrate in the diet must be controlled or drugs may be needed to stimulate the pancreas to produce more insulin or lower the blood glucose levels. Insulin may or may not be needed. Diabetes can occur in PREGNANCY and sometimes (but not always) disappears again after DELIVERY. Some doctors believe that pregnancy can reveal an already existing disease, but others consider it a separate form of diabetes, called Type III or gestational diabetes.

Diabetic women who are pregnant need careful monitoring to keep a close check on their condition, and they are normally considered a HIGH-RISK PREGNANCY. Good control of the diabetes during the first TRIMESTER of pregnancy greatly lowers the risk of abnormalities in the baby. If maternal blood sugar levels rise, the excess crosses the PLACENTA and is converted into muscles, fat and enlarged organs in the baby. The baby can be overweight and produces large quantities of insulin to cope with the high sugar level. When the baby is cut off from this at birth, it experiences a sudden, severe reduction in sugar while still producing large quantities of insulin. If this is not recognized and treated, the baby can suffer profound shortage of blood sugar (HYPOGLYCAEMIA), which can result in coma and death, and good ANTENATAL CARE is even more essential to prevent this from arising. The baby may also suffer from RESPIRATORY DISTRESS SYNDROME. The baby may additionally suffer mild hypoxia (shortage of oxygen to the tissues just prior to birth), and this can lead to neonatal JAUNDICE, which is easily treated. A diabetic mother may be more prone to urinary tract and other infections, THRUSH, high BLOOD PRESSURE, PRE-ECLAMPSIA, HYDRAMNIOS (excess amniotic fluid) and ECLAMPSIA. Delivery may be more difficult because of the large size of the baby, and FORCEPS may be needed, and the risk of STILLBIRTH is greater. Despite this, most diabetic women deliver vaginally and successfully. AMNIOCENTESIS may be carried out, and LABOUR may be induced if the baby's lungs are sufficiently mature, if problems have arisen. After delivery, the mother's insulin dosage must be carefully controlled until her body returns to normal.

diagnosis the process whereby a particular disease or condition is identified, based on simple observation, laboratory studies and tests using special equipment. The patient's medical history is very important. Laboratory tests on BLOOD, URINE, cerebrospinal fluid, semen, sputum or faeces may be needed as well as electrocardiographs or electroencephalographs to measure heart and brain activity respectively. Investigative techniques such as X-RAYS, MAMMOGRAPHY, THERMOGRAPHY, ULTRASOUND, COLPOSCOPY and exploratory LAPAROSCOPY may all be done. Body scans use radioactive substances and computers to build up a 3-D image of the body tissues and are good for diagnosing malignant tumours and other diseases affecting soft tissues. Types of body scans include computerized tomography (CT), nucleur magnetic resonance (NMI), Single Photon Emission Computed Tomography (SPECT) and Positron Emission Tomography (PET), each of which works best in particular tissue studies. In many instances the diagnosis requires greater skill than the treatment.

diaphragm (a) a membrane of muscle and tendon that separates the abdominal and chest cavities. (b) a BARRIER METHOD of CONTRACEPTION. The diaphragm is a dome of rubber with a flexible metal ring in its rim, which fits over the CERVIX. It is made in different sizes and types to fit women's shapes and must be properly fitted by a doctor. The fit should be checked each year, after childbirth, ABORTION, or a WEIGHT GAIN or loss of 10–15 pounds. The diaphragm is smeared with SPERMICIDE and inserted into the VAGINA and must be properly fitted each time to work properly. The diaphragm should not be inserted more than 2 hours before SEXUAL INTERCOURSE and the spermicide needs to be left in place for 8 hours to work. Fresh spermicide should be added for each act of intercourse. The diaphragm has a theoretical effectiveness of 97 per cent but actual figures are nearer to 85–90 per cent. The diaphragm should not be left in place for longer than 24 hours and on removal should be washed with soap and water, rinsed and dried. It should regularly be checked for holes and with care will last for around 2 years. Some women find a diaphragm irritates the URETHRA, causing URETHRITIS or CYSTITIS. This method of BIRTH CONTROL is currently increasing in popularity.

diarrhoea increased frequency and looseness of bowel movement, involving the passage of unusually soft faeces. Diarrhoea can be caused by food poisoning, colitis, irritable bowel syndrome, dysentery, etc. A severe case will result in the loss of water and salts that

must be replaced, and anti-diarrhoea drugs are used in certain circumstances.

dilatation and curettage *see* D AND C.

dilatation and evacuation (D and E) a procedure that combines a
D AND C with VACUUM ASPIRATION. It is mainly used as a method of
aborting a PREGNANCY of 12–18 weeks from the last menstrual period. Theoretically it can be used up to 24 weeks but is rarely performed as the CERVIX has to dilate too much in too short a time.
The longer the pregnancy the wider the cervix has to open to allow
access to instruments to remove the contents of the UTERUS. It can
be carried out under general or regional anaesthetic, and the tissue
is removed using a vacuum curette and suction. A curette is used to
make sure all the tissue is removed. Most doctors give the patient
OXYTOCIN to promote uterine CONTRACTIONS, which limits BLOOD loss
and returns the UTERUS to its normal pre-pregnant size. The operation takes 15–45 minutes, and an overnight stay in hospital is usually needed. There are fewer risks of complication than with induction methods of ABORTION, but INFECTION may still occur, causing
FEVER, VOMITING excessive bleeding and foul-smelling vaginal discharge requiring further treatment.

donor egg a method of ASSISTED CONCEPTION using an EGG produced
by a friend, relative or an anonymous donor. An EMBRYO is produced by fertilizing it with a SPERM, either artificially or IN VITRO.
The resulting embryo is transplanted to the UTERUS, and PREGNANCY
may result. Eggs can be taken from women who are having a
LAPAROSCOPY for TUBAL LIGATION by aspiration from an OVARY. Most
donors are given HORMONE injections for about a week prior to har-
vesting, which increase the number of eggs produced in one MEN-
STRUAL CYCLE to 4 or more. Donors are normally screened in various ways before eggs are retrieved. For women who have a functional uterus but do not ovulate, donor eggs may enable them to
become pregnant and have their partner's baby. Egg donation is
opposed by some religious groups, and there are legal and ethical
arguments that may cause problems in the future.

douching the rinsing of the VAGINA with warm water. It is thought
by some to be a means of preventing PREGNANCY but is not reliable.

SPERM can move through the cervical canal within 1–2 minutes after ejaculation and can reach the FALLOPIAN TUBES in 10 minutes. The pressure of the douching liquid can, in fact, speed up movement of sperm into the UTERUS. Douching disrupts the natural acidic environment of the vagina and can encourage the growth and spread of organisms that cause INFECTION. Douching is not necessary for good HYGIENE and should never be carried out if PREGNANCY is suspected or established, after a D AND C or ABORTION (for 2 weeks) or for 4–6 weeks after childbirth. It should not be carried out within 3 days of a GYNAECOLOGICAL EXAMINATION as it may make it more difficult to diagnose and treat an infection.

Down's syndrome a congenital or BIRTH DEFECT that is usually caused by the presence of an extra CHROMOSOME 21, so that there are 47 chromosomes in each body cell instead of the normal 46. People affected may suffer intellectual impairment, poor muscle tone, retarded growth, and have a small flat nose and slanting eyes (once termed 'mongolism'). Short, broad hands, a large tongue and protruding lower lip are further characteristics. About half of those with it have a congenital heart defect, and other characteristics are present to varying degrees. In most cases, the extra chromosome originates from the maternal egg, but it can arise from the father's sperm (33 per cent). Other genetic factors account for a rare 3 per cent of Down's syndrome births.

Down's syndrome is the most common congenital chromosome abnormality, occurring in 1 in every 600 to 800 births, but the true incidence is probably higher as many affected foetuses are believed to be spontaneously aborted in early PREGNANCY. Until quite recently, Down's syndrome children were unlikely to survive into adulthood and were confined in institutions. It is now recognized that those affected vary greatly in their degree of intellectual ability, just like normal children, and, given the correct stimulation, support and encouragement, can make very good progress. Treatment of Down's syndrome children has undergone a radical change so that early stimulation, nursery education and mainstream schooling are becoming more widely accepted. Some severely affected children still need care in a special unit, and others may require extra help with ordinary skills. Many go on to lead a fairly independent life in their community, requiring varying degrees of support. As with all children, parental love, encouragement and praise bring the greatest rewards and results.

The incidence of Down's syndrome is strongly correlated with maternal age, varying from 1 in 2000 births at age 20 to 1 in 100 at age 40. The risk of any chromosome abnormality arising is greatly increased in mothers over 35. AMNIOCENTESIS or CHORIONIC VILLUS SAMPLING are normally offered to older mothers, especially if there is any family history of chromosome abnormality in either parent. The cause of Down's syndrome is not known, but it seems that women's eggs are adversely affected by ageing. Abdominal X-RAYS, viral epidemics and incidence of infectious HEPATITIS appear to be correlated with a greater risk of Down's syndrome. Research is ongoing, and, in general, attitudes are gradually becoming more enlightened towards people with Down's syndrome. (*See also* CHROMOSOME TESTING; GENETIC SCREENING).

drug use in pregnancy nearly all substances ingested by a pregnant woman may move across the PLACENTA and have some effect on the child she is carrying. These include tobacco smoke, ALCOHOL, prescription and over-the-counter drugs, e.g. aspirin, paracetamol, laxatives and illegal substances. Hence, most medical authorities believe that no drug should be used at any stage of PREGNANCY (or BREAST-FEEDING) unless it is absolutely essential, and then in the smallest dose and for the shortest time period. Some drugs can be addictive both for mother and baby. A baby born to an addicted mother may be dependent on drugs and experience withdrawal symptoms. Some TRANQUILLIZERS have been found to cause death or damage to embryos in animal tests, and THALIDOMIDE is a tragic human example. Aspirin can disrupt the blood-clotting mechanism in the baby and the mother, and laxatives can interfere with the absorption of nutrients. Some antibiotics damage a developing FOETUS. Tetracycline is known to disrupt liver function in the baby and causes permanent discoloration of the teeth. Avoiding all drugs and remedies that may be hazardous is advisable during pregnancy, and a woman should always seek medical advice.

Duke's test a BLOOD test that is carried out to determine if a woman has developed ANTIBODIES against her partner's SPERM and therefore cannot conceive.

dysmenorrhoea pain and emotional discomfort associated with menstrual periods. This condition affects about a third of all women at some stage, and there are two types. Primary dysmenorrhoea occurs within 3 years of starting monthly periods, and there are CRAMPS and pains that are often severe enough to require bed rest. Other symptoms include NAUSEA, VOMITING, sweating, DIARRHOEA, pelvic soreness, and pain in the back and thighs. This form is most common in the under-25 age group, but it may continue into the mid-thirties and also after childbirth. Secondary dysmenorrhoea normally results from an underlying condition such as FIBROIDS, PELVIC INFLAMMATORY DISEASE, ENDOMETRIOSIS or the presence of an INTRAUTERINE DEVICE. Both types are thought to be caused by HORMONES called PROSTAGLANDINS, some of which cause uterine CONTRACTIONS. Excessive production of these hormones and/or sensitivity to them results in the painful menstrual cramps that occur. The condition can be relieved by bed rest with a hot water bottle, a hot bath, relaxation and some yoga exercises, and massage. Homoeopathic remedies, warm herbal teas (camomile, raspberry or mint), an alcoholic drink, or exercise such as aerobics or tennis can ease the pain. Drugs such as aspirin, ibuprofen or mefenamic acid all act as anti-prostaglandins and relieve the cramps and pain. The ORAL CONTRACEPTIVE PILL may be recommended to stop severe cramps, but this may have drawbacks and cannot be used by all women. The PROGESTERONE-releasing intrauterine device may also put a halt to period cramps.

dyspareunia painful vaginal intercourse. This can result from a local genital problem or be due to pain deep in the PELVIS. Pain in the VAGINA can result from irritation from a SPERMICIDE or from the rubber in a CONDOM or DIAPHRAGM, or a vaginal INFECTION such as THRUSH or TRICHOMONAS. Conditions such as PRURITIS VULVAE, HAEMORRHOIDS, urinary tract infections, painful perineal scar following EPISIOTOMY, and VAGINAL ATROPHY because of hormonal imbalance after childbirth, or the MENOPAUSE can all cause pain. Pain deep in the pelvis may be due to a prolapsed UTERUS, ENDOMETRIOSIS, PELVIC INFLAMMATORY DISEASE or other pelvic infection or result from a lack of lubricating fluid during penetration. These infections can usually be treated and cleared up easily, but a prolapsed uterus may need surgery. Women with little sexual experience may be afraid and tense up, leading to pain and lack of lubrication, which can exacerbate the problem. Pain during sex frequently has an emotional or psychological base. If a woman has had a bad sexual experience she is often afraid, and guilt, fear and shame can block her ability to enjoy sex and make the process painful. Here counselling and a sympathetic partner can help reveal the underlying problems so that they can be dealt with.

dysplasia in general, any abnormal development of tissues or organs. In women this normally refers to abnormalities in the cells of the CERVIX and UTERUS. These abnormalities may or may not be PRECANCEROUS LESIONS, and some doctors leave them to heal spontaneously while others recommend surgery.

The surface of the cervix consists of several layers that are constantly growing and replacing old cells. New cells grow in the basal layer and move to the top, maturing as they do so. When precancerous changes happen this process is disrupted and more immature cells are found on the surface of the cervix, often being large or malformed. The cervix may appear to have white patches on it (leukoplakia), have a red raised appearance or it may look no different from normal. It is the surface cells that are sampled in a CERVICAL SMEAR TEST, and the degree of dysplasia depends on the proportion of immature cells in the top layers of the cervix. When there are few mature cells in the top layer the condition is called CANCER in situ, which is localized and without invasive properties. In CERVICAL CANCER there are no mature cells in the top layer. If dysplasia is found in a smear test, the DIAGNOSIS is normally confirmed by COLPOSCOPY. If required, the abnormal cells are destroyed by CRYOSURGERY, CAUTERIZATION or LASER SURGERY. This usually cures the dysplasia, but it may recur. Surgical treatment, if needed, is in the form of a CONE BIOPSY or HYSTERECTOMY. Dysplasia can result from INFECTION, HORMONE therapy, ORAL CONTRACEPTIVES, radiation, emotional STRESS, environmental pollutants or any combination of these factors. Dysplasia rarely results in pain.

dystocia difficult LABOUR or childbirth, possibly caused by ABNORMAL PRESENTATION of the baby, an obstruction, a small BIRTH CANAL or uterine dysfunction (weak uterine CONTRACTIONS). (*See also* PROLONGED LABOUR.)

dysuria painful urination. This is normally the result of a bacterial INFECTION in the BLADDER or kidneys or an obstruction of the urinary tract, e.g. urinary calculus (stone). (*See also* CYSTITIS).

E

eclampsia an ACUTE condition that is life-threatening to both mother and FOETUS. It generally occurs after 24 weeks of PREGNANCY or just after childbirth and is characterized by grand mal convulsions, coma, HYPERTENSION, OEDEMA and protein in the URINE. The condition is normally preceded by PRE-ECLAMPSIA, which can often be controlled so that eclampsia does not develop. Symptoms of eclampsia are HEADACHE, ANXIETY, blurred vision, high pulse rate, exaggerated reflex, high temperature and decreased urinary output. In eclampsia, the BLOOD vessels of the UTERUS go into spasm and cut down the blood flow to the foetus. This can cause low levels of oxygen in the tissues and foetal death. The foetus may also die because of drugs used to treat maternal convulsions, or because of injury or damage during LABOUR, or because it is too PREMATURE to survive. DELIVERY is usually by means of CAESAREAN SECTION. The woman's condition then usually improves within a couple of days, but occasionally the convulsions resume and can be severe or even fatal. Convulsions may only develop after delivery in some cases and can be mild, moderate or severe, possibly leading to death. Treatment aims to stop convulsions, reduce BLOOD PRESSURE, increase blood flow and sedate the brain. Delivery of the baby, by Caesarean section, also helps to improve the condition. The cause of both pre-eclampsia and eclampsia is unknown. Around 50 per cent of all cases develop before delivery (mainly in the last TRIMESTER), 25 per cent during labour and 25 per cent after delivery (normally within 24 hours). Eclampsia is 3 times more common in first pregnancies and 4 times more common in MULTIPLE PREGNANCIES. It is also associated with ECTOPIC PREGNANCY and a HYDATIDIFORM MOLE, and a woman whose mother had eclampsia is more likely to develop the condition. If a woman has had eclampsia once, she is far more likely to develop it again in subsequent pregnancies. (*See also* HYPERTENSION).

ectopic pregnancy a PREGNANCY that develops in an organ other than the UTERUS. The most common site is in the FALLOPIAN TUBE (99 per cent), but rarely the fertilized egg implants in an OVARY, the abdominal or pelvic cavity or in the cervical canal. FERTILIZATION of an EGG by a SPERM normally occurs in the Fallopian tube, from where the egg travels down the tube to the uterus. If the tube is damaged or blocked, however, this process cannot take place, and the egg remains in the tube. The Fallopian tubes can be damaged because of ENDOMETRIOSIS, PELVIC INFLAMMATORY DISEASE, past or present use of an INTRAUTERINE DEVICE, GONORRHOEA, or some other disorder. One in 100 pregnancies is ectopic, and they are more common in first pregnancies, after using EMERGENCY POST-COITAL CONTRACEPTION and in women taking the PROGESTERONE-only MINIPILL.

There are two forms of ectopic pregnancy: subacute and ACUTE. The subacute form causes abdominal and referred shoulder PAIN, usually on only one side, possible vaginal bleeding, and FAINTING. There may have been at least one missed menstrual period, but a PREGNANCY TEST is not always positive. The subacute form is usually detected after 8–10 weeks GESTATION before rupture of the Fallopian tube. It may be treated by injecting into the embryo a toxic substance that causes it to die, the tissue being reabsorbed into the woman's body and the Fallopian tube preserved. In other cases, surgery to remove the embryo and tube may be needed. The acute form is not diagnosed until the tube ruptures, which causes severe pain and shock, HAEMORRHAGE, dizziness, pallor, faintness and low BLOOD PRESSURE. This is an emergency that needs immediate hospitalization for surgical removal (and the ovary may need to be taken out as well). Sometimes the embryo can be removed, leaving the

Fallopian tube. The remaining Fallopian tube is normally intact but needs to be checked as it may be affected by the condition that brought about the ectopic pregnancy. A HYSTERECTOMY may be required if irrevocable damage has occurred and future pregnancy is impossible. Ectopic pregnancy can be detected using ULTRASOUND, and a woman's risk significantly increases in a subsequent pregnancy, since the underlying infection or condition may still be present. Sixty per cent of women who have had ectopic pregnancies become pregnant again, 30 per cent avoid pregnancy voluntarily and 10 per cent become infertile. Numbers are increasing in developed countries, and this may relate to improved detection techniques.

eczema INFLAMMATION of the skin that causes ITCHING, a red rash and often small blisters that weep and become encrusted. This may be followed by the skin thickening and then peeling off in scales. There are several types of eczema, atopic being the most common. (Atopic is the hereditary tendency to develop allergic reactions because of an ANTIBODY in the skin.) It is often the case that eczema, asthma and hay fever are all found in the family history, but many children with eczema from a young age improve markedly as they approach the age of 10 or 11. Treatment usually involves steroid creams.

effacement a process in which the cervical canal becomes thinner and shorter during the last month of PREGNANCY and the first stage of LABOUR. It converts the tube-like cervical canal into a wide funnel. BRAXTON-HICK CONTRACTIONS ensure much of the effacement takes place before labour begins, and many women are 80 per cent effaced by the time this starts.

egg the female reproductive cell found in all sexually reproducing animals, including humans. Eggs are present in the ovaries of girls at birth but mature and start to be released only during PUBERTY. At birth the ovaries contain 300,000 eggs, by age 12 there are 75,000, and after the MENOPAUSE no eggs remain. An egg survives outside the ovary for around 24 hours before it degenerates. The latin term is ovum. (*See also* OVULATION; MENSTRUAL CYCLE).

embolism a blockage of an ARTERY by an embolus, which obstructs

BLOOD flow. An embolus can be a BLOOD CLOT, fat, an air bubble, amniotic fluid or a foreign body. One of the most dangerous types of embolism is pulmonary embolism, in which a blood clot, originating in a deep VEIN in the leg or PELVIS, travels and lodges in an artery supplying the lungs. This may be fatal and is a complication of DEEP-VEIN THROMBOSIS. A systemic embolism is caused by an embolus in any other artery and can develop after a heart attack. Gangrene can arise if a limb is involved or a STROKE if the embolism affects the brain. Treatment takes the form of anticoagulant drugs to thin the blood and drugs to dissolve the embolus. (*See also* ARTERIOSCLEROSIS; PHLEBITIS).

embryo an organism in the early stages of development. In human beings it refers to the period of development between IMPLANTATION in the UTERUS (which occurs about 2 weeks after CONCEPTION) until the end of the 7th or 8th week of GESTATION. After this time the embryo is called a FOETUS.

embryo transfer *see* ASSISTED CONCEPTION; IN VITRO FERTILIZATION

emergency contraception or **postcoital contraception** CONTRACEPTION used after unprotected SEXUAL INTERCOURSE or when there is reason to suspect that the usual method has failed (e.g. a CONDOM bursting). There are two methods: a special dose of the combined contraceptive pill and an INTRAUTERINE DEVICE. Both work by stopping an EMBRYO from implanting into the lining of the UTERUS, and, while highly effective, neither is infallible in preventing PREGNANCY.

The true degree of effectiveness is difficult to gauge as some women may already have an unsuspected pregnancy when they seek this form of contraception. It is, however, in the order of 95 per cent for the emergency pill and almost 100 per cent for the IUD. Both are normally available from the usual outlets, i.e. GPs' surgeries, family planning and genito-urinary clinics. The pill is a special formulation of two tablets, the second taken 12 hours after the first, and must be started within 72 hours of unprotected intercourse. A woman may feel NAUSEA or actually vomit (because of the high dose of OESTROGEN in the preparation), and if this occurs, a replacement pill must be taken. The postcoital pill can be taken by women who would not normally be prescribed combined oral contraceptives because of the presence of some risk factor. Although it contains a high dose of oestrogen, it is safe if only taken occasionally but should not be used frequently or more than once in any MENSTRUAL CYCLE.

An IUD should be fitted within five days, or 120 hours, of unprotected intercourse, and it may be removed once a menstrual period has occurred, or continued with as a permanent means of contraception.

endocrine glands ductless GLANDS that secrete HORMONES and other substances directly into the bloodstream (or LYMPH). The main endocrine glands are the PANCREAS, PITUITARY, THYROID, parathyroid, HYPOTHALAMUS, PINEAL GLAND, ADRENAL glands, ovaries (and testes in males), and the PLACENTA. Together they make up the endocrine system, and all are influenced by one another. Their secretory capability is interlinked, and this controls many body functions including reproduction. The interdependent relationship between the glands results in the changes in endocrine activity that happen at PUBERTY, CONCEPTION, PREGNANCY and the MENOPAUSE.

endometrial cancer a rare type of CANCER, which is a MALIGNANT growth of cells in the lining of the UTERUS, the ENDOMETRIUM. PRECANCEROUS growths in the endometrium may be present for many years before becoming malignant. Endometrial cancer is more common in postmenopausal women, and 75 per cent of sufferers are over 50. Conditions that increase the risk of developing this disease are OBESITY, a family history of endometrial cancer, HYPERTENSION and DIABETES. Women who have not had children or those who were exposed to diethylstilbestrol (DES) while in the uterus have a higher risk of endometrial cancer. Symptoms include abnormal vaginal bleeding, either between periods or after SEXUAL INTERCOURSE, POSTMENOPAUSAL BLEEDING, cramping pains in the abdomen, vaginal discharge and increased frequency of urination caused by the tumour pressing on the BLADDER. Investigations may involve ULTRASOUND, but normally a D AND C is needed to check the endometrium for growths. Examination of tissue samples identifies cancerous cells, and then a total HYSTERECTOMY with removal of the UTERUS, FALLOPIAN TUBES and ovaries is usually needed and, possibly, RADIOTHERAPY, to destroy any stray malignant cells. If the cancer has spread outside the uterus, more radical surgery may be needed to remove the top of the VAGINA and the GLANDS of the PELVIS. If the cancer is detected early on, there is a high rate of cure (up to 90 per cent) with SURGERY and radiotherapy. As the disease spreads, the cure rate drops to around 40 per cent. (*See also* UTERINE CANCER).

endometrial resection and abalation a relatively new surgical procedure in which the ENDOMETRIUM or lining of the WOMB is completely removed using an electric current (diathermy) or laser beam (*compare* D AND C) It is carried out to correct heavy menstrual bleeding and makes subsequent periods very light. PREGNANCY is unlikely following this procedure but is still possible. A hormonal injection to thin the endometrium is needed about 5 weeks before the operation, which is carried out under general anaesthetic. It is considered to be an effective treatment when the only symptom is heavy bleeding, requiring an overnight stay in hospital and quick return to normal life.

endometriosis a condition in which endometrial tissue grows outside the UTERUS in abnormal sites. These include the outside of the WOMB itself, ovaries, FALLOPIAN TUBES, BLADDER, bowel and other areas in the PELVIS. The tissue may even be found in the lungs, PANCREAS, kidneys and eyes. If this tissue penetrates the wall of the uterus, the resulting condition is called adenomyosis. Although not in its natural site, the endometrial tissue reacts to HORMONES, which control reproduction as if it were in situ. Early in the cycle, as OESTROGEN is produced, the tissue fills with BLOOD and swells. During the MENSTRUAL CYCLE the tissue breaks down and bleeds, and the blood is trapped in the pelvic cavity (or elsewhere), eventually forming a CYST. The patches of tissue also cause INFLAMMATION and scar tissue formation, which is repeated month after month, leading to ADHESIONS. Symptoms of this condition are DYSMENORRHOEA, pain (possibly severe) during intercourse and menstrual cramps that become more acute on the last day of the period, and reduced FERTILITY or even INFERTILITY if the Fallopian tubes are affected. There may also be PELVIC and BACK PAIN and also in urination (DYSURIA) and on moving the bowels. About 75 per cent of cases are in women between 25 and 45, but it can affect any age group from MENARCHE to the MENOPAUSE. The pain from endometriosis may be so severe as to be completely disabling and can prevent enjoyment of a normal life.

Diagnosis is difficult and requires LAPAROSCOPY or other exploratory surgery. The cysts and adhesions may be difficult to locate. Cysts change in both colour and size throughout the menstrual cycle. They vary from a pinhead to a walnut in size and may be few or up to 100 can be present. Treatment is aimed at stopping menstruation. Endometriosis ceases during pregnancy and may not recur afterwards. ORAL CONTRACEPTIVES can help control the condition, but the most common drug used is danazol, a type of hormone therapy that acts on the PITUITARY gland to stop OVULATION and menstruation. Side-effects include WEIGHT GAIN, ACNE, oily skin and hair growth. The drug Nafarelin also acts to suppress ovulation and menstruation and is administered as a nasal spray. It too has side-effects, similar to those of the menopause, i.e. HOT FLUSHES, vaginal dryness and decreased sex drive. Both drugs are temporary treatments, and almost half the women with this condition are unable to conceive. Mild forms of it can interrupt FERTILIZATION or IMPLANTATION, and some doctors believe that the body produces ANTIBODIES against the stray endometrial tissue, which attack the uterine lining itself. This may explain the high rates of MISCARRIAGE in women with endometriosis (3 times the normal rate). The greater risk of ECTOPIC PREGNANCY (16 per cent) that occurs may be due to damage to the Fallopian tubes caused by scar tissue or adhesions. Removal of patches of endometrial tissue can be done with LASER SURGERY or CAUTERIZATION, and cysts can be removed from the ovaries, allowing them to function normally. HYSTERECTOMY may be considered as a final option if the woman has completed her family and hormone treatment has not helped. Endometriosis tends to get progressively worse throughout life, until the menopause when the condition usually declines.

endometritis INFLAMMATION and INFECTION of the ENDOMETRIUM. Symptoms are pelvic pain, a thick, yellowish vaginal discharge that

may be foul smelling and a tender UTERUS (upon PELVIC EXAMINA-
TION). The condition may occur because of irritation by an INTRAU-
TERINE DEVICE or as a complication of a first-trimester ABORTION.
The inflammation can be cleared by antibiotics.

endometrium a MUCOUS MEMBRANE that lines the UTERUS and consists of several layers. It varies in thickness throughout the MEN-
STRUAL CYCLE, gradually being built up in preparation for PREG-
NANCY. If FERTILIZATION does not occur, most of the endometrium
is lost in the MENSTRUAL FLOW. After MENOPAUSE, the whole endometrium wastes away. It can develop a range of conditions (*see*
ENDOMETRIAL CANCER; POLYPS; ENDOMETRIOSIS).

engagement a descent of the baby's head into the PELVIS shortly before birth. It can occur from 36 weeks onwards but may not take
place until the second stage of LABOUR, when the CERVIX is fully
dilated. In most first-time mothers, engagement occurs in the last
few weeks of PREGNANCY, and it shows that the pelvic inlet is large
enough for the baby. Engagement reduces the pressure on the woman's lungs as the baby 'drops' or moves down, so breathing may be
easier, but pressure on the bladder tends to increase. It is popularly
known as 'lightening'.

epidural anaesthetic a type of regional ANAESTHETIA that is commonly used in LABOUR, CAESAREAN SECTION and TUBAL LIGATION. A
local anaesthetic is injected into the epidural space—the area around
the spinal cord inside the vertebral column. This blocks pain from
the waist to the knees but allows motor nerve function so CONTRAC-
TIONS can continue. It can be administered fairly early in labour
and maintained until DELIVERY by additional doses of anaesthetic.
An epidural continued during the second stage of labour means
the urge to push is not usually felt, and a woman may need to be
directed to do so by the MIDWIFE or doctor. An epidural anaesthetic
lowers BLOOD PRESSURE, which is beneficial for women with HYPER-
TENSION, PRE-ECLAMPSIA or ECLAMPSIA, and it reduces the work required from muscles and organs, which aids women with DIABETES
or any heart or lung condition. However, there are some disadvantages. The procedure is difficult to carry out and needs a skilled
anaesthetist, but in some cases may not block all nerves. Incorrect

positioning of the needle (which may happen if the woman inadvertently moves) can allow anaesthetic to leak into the spinal fluid, which causes a drop in the mother's blood pressure and is dangerous to her and the baby. An epidural often slows down labour, and EPISIOTOMY and FORCEPS are more likely to be needed. Despite these difficulties, it is the most commonly used type of regional anaesthesia and is helpful for many women.

episiotomy a surgical procedure in which the PERINEUM is cut to enlarge the vaginal opening, carried out in DELIVERY normally during the second stage of LABOUR as the baby's head is crowning. A local ANAESTHETIC is injected into the perineum and an incision is made towards the anus. After birth, the cut is stitched, and the stitches may either dissolve or fall out after a few weeks.. Episiotomy is carried out if a rapid delivery is desirable, e.g. if there is foetal distress. Also, if the baby's head is too large for the vaginal opening, if FORCEPS or VENTOUSE DELIVERY methods are used or if the baby is BREECH. A birth in which the perineum hasn't had time to stretch sufficiently because of a quick labour, or if pushing has occurred too soon, often requires an episiotomy. Also, one may be needed if the mother has become exhausted.

The need for this procedure is lessened if natural childbirth positions are used (upright or on all fours) as these allow the perineal tissues to thin gradually. Also, controlling the baby's head and allowing it to come out of the vaginal opening between contractions, and perineal massage, can help to thin the tissue and reduce tearing. Recent evidence has shown that tears in the perineum heal faster and with less pain than episiotomy cuts. Episiotomy is common in the western world, but some people now consider it unnecessary surgery. Women may have problems with episiotomy stitches and scars, but also with natural tears. Stitches can be painful when sitting down or going to the toilet. Warm baths, ice packs or sitting on a rubber ring can help ease the initial discomfort. In some cases discomfort can prevent resumption of sexual relations and have long-term adverse physical and emotional effects.

exercise physical exertion that is important for many aspects of physical and mental health. Regular exercise is important throughout life as it improves BLOOD circulation and muscle tone, enlarges lung capacity, aids bowel function and the digestive system, lowers body weight, promotes good posture and RELAXATION, and encourages good sleeping patterns. Exercise reduces the chances of developing a heart attack, angina and other HEART DISEASE, STROKE, backache, DIABETES, HYPERTENSION, and GALLSTONES. The risk of CANCER of the ENDOMETRIUM, colon, BREAST, CERVIX and OVARY are less in active people.

Exercise can increase BONE density, which is important in postmenopausal women in lessening the adverse effects of OSTEOPOROSIS. It can alsoboost energy levels and improve a person's mood, reduce FATIGUE and tension, and may lessen PREMENSTRUAL TENSION and period pain. In addition, exercises for strength, suppleness and stamina can considerably improve life expectancy and vigour in older age. If a person has a special medical condition, is over-weight or a smoker, she should consult a doctor for advice on suitable forms of exercise.

F

fainting a temporary, brief loss of consciousness caused by a sudden drop in the BLOOD supply to the brain. It can occur in perfectly healthy people, brought about by prolonged standing or emotional shock. It may also occur during PREGNANCY or result from an INFECTION or from severe pain or loss of blood through injury. It is often preceded by giddiness, blurred vision, sweating and ringing in the ears. Recovery is usually complete, producing no lasting illeffects, although this depends on the underlying cause.

Fallopian tubes a pair of tubes, one leading from each OVARY to the WOMB. At the ovary, the tube is expanded to form a funnel with finger-like projections, known as fimbriae, surrounding the opening. This funnel does not communicate directly with the ovary but is open to the abdominal cavity. When an EGG is released from the ovary, however, the fimbriae move and waft it into the Fallopian tube. The tube is about 10–12cm long and leads directly into the womb at the lower end through a narrow opening. The main function of the Fallopian tubes is to provide an environment in which the SPERM and egg can combine, eventually to produce an EMBRYO. Sometimes the Fallopian tube fails to move a fertilized egg into the uterus, and IMPLANTATION takes place in the wall, producing an ECTOPIC PREGNANCY.

Proper functioning of the Fallopian tubes is necessary for CONCEPTION, and scarring of them is the most common cause of female INFERTILITY. This can occur as a result of ENDOMETRIOSIS, previous ectopic pregnancy, bowel surgery, PELVIC INFLAMMATORY DISEASE, gynaecological surgery, INFECTION after childbirth or ADHESIONS because of abdominal surgery. Laser or microsurgery may be able to repair the damage in some cases. Tying of the Fallopian tubes prevents CONCEPTION and is surgically performed in female STERILIZATION. The tubes may become inflamed or infected (SALPINGITIS), and this can have several causes. CANCER of the Fallopian tubes is rare and can be related to malignancy in the UTERUS or ovaries. Surgical removal of the Fallopian tubes may be necessary in HYSTERECTOMY or removal of an ectopic pregnancy. (*See also* SALPINGECTOMY; TUBAL LIGATION.)

false labour irregular CONTRACTIONS of the UTERUS that are mistaken for true LABOUR when a PREGNANCY is near full term. They can occur throughout pregnancy but are different from those in labour as they are not regular, have variable frequency and do not become progressively stronger. The only way to distinguish between true and false labour is examination of the CERVIX to see if dilation is taking place. (*See also* BRAXTON-HICK CONTRACTIONS.)

false pregnancy a condition in which a woman has signs of PREGNANCY such as WEIGHT GAIN, AMENORRHOEA, MORNING SICKNESS and breast enlargement but without CONCEPTION taking place. It can be an emotional or psychological condition in which a woman wishes to conceive but cannot do so, or may be due to an extreme fear of pregnancy. It may also be caused by a tumour or disfunction of the ENDOCRINE system.

family planning the use of CONTRACEPTION to limit or plan when children are born to a particular couple. Family planning is avail-

able in hospital clinics or at GPs' surgeries. (*See also* BIRTH CON-
TROL; ABORTION.)

fatigue physical and mental tiredness that may be a symptom of illness or result from too much activity and too little sleep. It is a
common complaint that can range from tiredness to exhaustion. It
can result from a THYROID GLAND disorder, INSOMNIA, inadequate
diet, ANAEMIA, PREGNANCY, DEPRESSION, ANXIETY or a heart condition. It may also be caused by DIABETES, some drugs MYALGIC EN-
CEPHALOMYELITIS (ME), ALCOHOL consumption, MENOPAUSE, viral
illnesses and CANCER. Prolonged fatigue needs to be investigated so
that the condition or reason causing the problem can be diagnosed
and treated.

fertility the ability to conceive and carry a child to term. A woman's
fertility is dependent on OVULATION, FALLOPIAN TUBES, the condition of the CERVICAL MUCUS, FERTILIZATION, EMBRYO IMPLANTATION
and maintenance of PREGNANCY. Fertility peaks in women in their
mid-twenties and declines slowly through the thirties, accelerating
in the forties. Fertility ends with the MENOPAUSE. (*See also* INFERTIL-
ITY).

fertilization the fusion of SPERM and EGG to form a ZYGOTE, which
then undergoes cell division to become an EMBRYO. In humans it
takes place high up in the FALLOPIAN TUBE near the OVARY, and the
fertilized egg travels down and becomes implanted in the WOMB.

fetoscopy a technique that allows the developing FOETUS and amniotic fluid to be viewed while still in the WOMB. It may be carried out
from the 15th to 20th week of PREGNANCY by inserting a special
instrument, called a fetoscope (a form of endoscope), through the
abdominal wall into the UTERUS. The foetus can be viewed and samples of BLOOD or tissue taken to determine if certain disorders or
defects are present. It is carried out under local anaesthetic, using
ULTRASOUND to monitor the baby's position. The procedure allows
DIAGNOSIS of physical defects of the limbs, eyes, GENITALS, ears,
mouth and spine, and detects the presence of MECONIUM in the
amniotic fluid, a sign of foetal distress. Blood disorders such as
SICKLE-CELL ANAEMIA, THALASSAEMIA or HAEMOPHILIA can be detected
with certainty. Some cases of sickle-cell anaemia are missed with

AMNIOCENTESIS. Examination of samples obtained by fetoscopy can also indicate the presence of toxic substances, VIRUSES or parasites, and the procedure may be used to administer medication to the foetus. Minor surgical procedures can be carried out *in utero* via a fetoscope. (*See also* CHORIONIC VILLUS SAMPLING.)

fetus *see* **foetus**.

fever an elevation of body temperature above the normal, which accompanies many diseases and INFECTIONS. Its cause is the production by the body of endogenous pyrogen, which acts on the thermoregulatory centre in the HYPOTHALAMUS in the brain. This responds by promoting mechanisms that increase heat generation and lessen heat loss, leading to a rise in temperature. Fever is the main factor in many infections caused by bacteria or VIRUSES and results from toxins produced by the growth of these organisms. Fevers are classed as specific, intermittent, remittent and relapsing, according to their causative agent. Treatment of fever depends on the underlying cause. It may be necessary to reduce the temperature by direct methods, such as sponging the body with tepid water, or by giving drugs such as aspirin. As well as a rise in body temperature, symptoms of fever include HEADACHE, NAUSEA, shivering, DIARRHOEA or CONSTIPATION. Above 40° C (105° F), there may be delirium or convulsions, especially in young children.

fibroadenoma a BENIGN lump in the BREAST that feels firm, rubbery and smooth with well-defined edges. It develops in a single breast lobule and is made up of excess connective and GLANDular tissue. Fibroadenomas are more common in women aged 15–35 and in black and oriental races. There appears to be a hereditary factor, and 20 per cent of women with this condition have more than one lump present in both breasts. The average number is 2–4 lumps. Fibroadenomas may not be diagnosed until after PREGNANCY or the MENOPAUSE, when lumps are easier to detect. They are normally closely monitored for growth or change, and a BIOPSY may be required. Surgery may be carried out to remove the lump, and this does not affect BREAST-FEEDING. In some European countries, treatment is by means of hormonal drugs such as danazol, PROGESTER-ONE and tamoxifen, but these can have unpleasant SIDE-EFFECTS.

Fibroadenomas often recur after surgery so treatment methods differ for individual women. A type of non-invasive CANCER can develop from a fibroadenoma, but this is extremely rare and easily treated. (*See also* MASTITIS; MASTALGIA.)

fibroid a BENIGN tumour of the ENDOMETRIUM that normally grows inside the UTERUS. They are very common, particularly in black women, and can range in size from a pea to a large grapefruit. Untreated fibroids may reach a weight in excess of 20 pounds. The growth of these tumours is stimulated by OESTROGEN, and hence PREGNANCY, the combined contraceptive pill and HORMONE REPLACEMENT THERAPY may contribute to their growth. Symptoms include heavy, painful and prolonged peiods, DYSURIA, CONSTIPATION, backache, discomfort during intercourse, swollen abdomen and a feeling of heaviness. Depending on their site, fibroids may exert pressure on the BLADDER or bowel, causing pain, but in some cases there are no symptoms present.

There are several different types of fibroid, each of which may cause specific problems. Fibroids may be detected during PELVIC EXAMINATION, HYSTEROSCOPY or ULTRASOUND investigation. A D AND C may be sufficient to remove small fibroids, but a myomectomy operation may be needed. This leaves the uterus intact but fibroids can regrow, and scar tissue and ADHESIONS may form. These can adversely affect FERTILITY and increase the risk of MISCARRIAGE. Fibroids can be removed by LAPAROSCOPY or hysteroscopy, drugs that stop oestrogen production being used first to shrink their size. These two surgical techniques cause less scarring and are not so likely to affect fertility adversely. If fibroids are very large and the woman's family is complete, a HYSTERECTOMY may be carried out. Fibroids can grow during pregnancy and may interfere with the PLACENTA, a situation requiring careful monitoring.

fistula an abnormal opening between two hollow organs or between such an organ or GLAND and the exterior. These may arise during development so that a baby may be born with a fistula. Alternatively, they can be produced by injury, INFECTION or as a complication following surgery.

fluid retention an accumulation of fluid in body tissues. It often appears as swelling of the ankles or hands, apparent WEIGHT GAIN and puffiness of the face or neck. Many women suffer from fluid retention before their menstrual period or during PREGNANCY. The reason for this is unclear, but it may be due to high levels of OES-TROGEN and PROGESTERONE in the body. Severe fluid retention is a symptom of several serious disorders, including liver, kidney or HEART DISEASE and ECLAMPSIA. It is treated by diuretic drugs that increase the flow of URINE and drain tissues. A reduction in the intake of salt in the diet is usually recommended. Swollen ankles can also result from prolonged standing (*see* VARICOSE VEINS).

foetal monitoring all techniques used to record the growth and development of a FOETUS through PREGNANCY, LABOUR and DELIVERY. External palpation of the mother's abdomen carried out during antenatal visits determines the size of the foetus and its position. The foetal heartbeat may be monitored by a sonic aid, stethoscope or electronic monitor. An ULTRASOUND scan is usually performed at least once to check development of the foetus. During labour, foetal heartbeat is monitored and can detect distress. The monitor can be strapped to the woman's abdomen, and this is becoming routine in most hospitals. Electronic foetal monitoring is used routinely in all HIGH-RISK pregnancies, if labour is induced or if an EPIDURAL is given. AMNIOCENTESIS, CHORIONIC VILLUS SAMPLING, ALPHA-FETOPROTEIN tests, UMBILICAL CORD SAMPLING and FETOSCOPY can also be considered as methods of foetal monitoring.

foetus or **fetus** a developing EMBRYO after the 8th week of GESTA-TION.

follicle, ovarian a small group of cells that surround an EGG in the OVARY. Every month follicle-stimulating hormone (FSH) produced by the PITUITARY GLAND stimulates several of the ovarian follicles to grow and produce OESTROGEN. Gradually all but one (or two) of the follicles degenerate, and the surviving one, then called the GRAA-FIAN FOLLICLE, matures under the influence of luteinizing hormone (LH). It moves to the surface of the OVARY, ruptures and releases an EGG (OVULATION). The cells of the follicle then form the CORPUS LU-TEUM, which produces the hormones oestrogen and PROGESTERONE. If the egg is not fertilized, hormone levels change and the corpus luteum degenerates. Occasionally the follicle does not disintegrate and forms an OVARIAN CYST.

follicle stimulating hormone *see* FSH.

forceps a surgical instrument used to assist and speed up the DELIVERY of a baby. They may be used during the second stage of LABOUR if there is maternal or foetal distress, the UMBILICAL CORD is around the baby's neck, there is an unusual presentation, PREMATURE BIRTH or a very long delivery. Forceps have been used since the late 16th century. (*See also* VENTOUSE DELIVERY.)

FSH (follicle-stimulating hormone) a HORMONE produced by the PITUITARY GLAND that stimulates the growth of FOLLICLES in the ovaries. It is partly responsible for the production of a mature EGG and the production of OESTROGEN from the ovaries. (*See also* OVULATION; MENSTRUAL CYCLE.)

G

galactocele a CYST in the BREAST that is caused by blockage of one of the milk-secreting GLANDS.

galactorrhoea a persistent flow of breast milk after PREGNANCY in a woman who is not BREAST-FEEDING or abnormal production in a non-pregnant woman. It is usually associated with AMENORRHOEA and often caused by a PITUITARY GLAND tumour. Other causes are hormonal imbalance, certain TRANQUILLIZER drugs and some ORAL CONTRACEPTIVE PILLS. Treatment depends on the cause but usually includes various drugs such as bromocriptine, surgical removal of a tumour and, occasionally, RADIOTHERAPY.

gall bladder a sac-like organ, situated on the underside of the liver, that stores and concentrates bile. It is approximately 8 cm long and 2.5 cm across at its widest point, and its volume is a little over 30 cubic cm. When fats are digested, the gall bladder contracts, sending bile into the duodenum through the common bile duct. GALLSTONES, the most common gall bladder disease, may form in certain circumstances. Other gall bladder diseases include fatty dyspepsia and cholecystitis (INFLAMMATION).

gallstones stones of varying composition that form in the GALL BLAD-
DER. Their formation seems to be caused by a change in bile composition, rendering CHOLESTEROL less soluble. Stones may also form
around a foreign body. There are three types of stone: cholesterol,
pigment and mixed, the last being the most common. Calcium salts
are usually found in varying proportions. Although gallstones may
be present for years without symptoms, they can cause severe pain
and may pass into the common bile duct to cause, by the resulting
obstruction, JAUNDICE.

gamete a mature germ or sexual cell, male or female, that can participate in FERTILIZATION, e.g. EGG and SPERM.

Gaucher's disease a hereditary disease in which an enzyme that
allows the body to break down and eliminate accumulations of certain fats in the cells is lacking. It is a recessive-GENE disorder similar to TAY-SACHS DISEASE and is most common in European Jewish
people. It causes fatty substances to build up in the spleen, liver
and BONE MARROW, which leads to enlargement of the organs, swollen joints and brittle bones. Progression differs from patient to patient, and if it appears in infancy is more severe and survival may
only be 1–2 years. The less ACUTE form arises later in life and has a
better outlook. The disease is incurable but is treated with enzyme
replacement therapy. Gaucher's disease can be detected in an AM-
NIOCENTESIS test. (*See also* BIRTH DEFECTS).

gene the fundamental unit of genetic material found at a specific
location on a CHROMOSOME. It is chemically complex and responsible for the transmission of information from older to younger gen-
erations. Each gene contributes to a particular trait or characteristic. There are more than 100,000 genes in humans, and size varies
with the characteristic, e.g. the gene that codes for the HORMONE
insulin is 1700 base pairs long. There are several types of gene,
depending on function, and in addition genes are said to be dominant or recessive. A dominant characteristic is one that occurs whenever the gene is present while the effect of a recessive gene (say a
disease) will be apparent only if it is present on both members of
the chromosome pair, i.e. it must be homo-zygous.

genetic code specific information carried by DNA molecules that controls the particular amino acids and their positions in every protein and thus all the proteins synthesized within a cell. Since there are just four NUCLEOTIDES, a unit of three bases becomes the smallest one that can produce codes for all 20 amino acids. The transfer of information from gene to protein is based on three consecutive nucleotides called codons. A change in the genetic code results in an amino acid being inserted incorrectly in a protein, resulting in a mutation.

genetic counselling professional counselling and advice aimed at determining a couple's risk of passing on a hereditary disorder to their child. It may be needed because a previous child has a chromosomal or genetic disorder or CONGENITAL DEFECT or if the partners are related. Advice may be offered if there is a history of repeated MISCARRIAGE or any family background of certain disorders.

A complete family and medical history is compiled and a series of laboratory tests may be performed, including metabolic, urinary and GENETIC SCREENING. Parents can then decide whether to attempt to conceive a child, based on the best possible medical knowledge and advice. Some estimates suggest that every individual carries 3–8 GENES for genetic defects and each couple has a 3 per cent chance of bearing a child with a BIRTH DEFECT.

genetic screening the procedure whereby individuals are tested to determine whether their genetic make-up suggests they carry a particular disease or condition. If it is shown that someone carries a genetically linked disease then decisions can be taken regarding future children.

genitals the male or female reproductive organs, often referring to the external parts only.

genital herpes a common disease that is caused by the HERPES simplex II VIRUS. It causes blisters on the VULVA, anus and possibly the upper thighs, with FEVER, and swollen GLANDS in the groin. There may be numbness of the vulva, which is sensitive to touch, and DYSURIA. It is more common in women as warm, moist conditions in the genital region favour INFECTION. It is highly contagious and can be spread to partners through sexual or other close contact, and the eyes may be affected. The disease is considered incurable as it cannot be eliminated from the body and goes through cycles of activity and dormancy. The blisters appear 3–20 days after infection and soon become painful. They can be treated with new antiviral agents, such as Zovirax, that shorten the attack and stop the spread of blisters. No medication can prevent a recurrence, and all sexual partners should be treated to limit a cycle of re-infection. If an active infection is diagnosed in the last TRIMESTER of PREGNANCY, a vaginal DELIVERY is not advised as the virus can be passed on to the baby, possibly causing brain damage and/or blindness. Genital herpes increases the risk of CERVICAL CANCER so regular CERVICAL SMEAR TESTS are particularly important. (*See also* CONGENITAL INFECTION).

genital warts another name for GENITAL HERPES.

German measles a highly infectious disease that mainly occurs in childhood and is caused by the rubella VIRUS. After a 2–3 week INCUBATION PERIOD symptoms of a slight FEVER, sore throat, shivering and HEADACHE appear. Then a rash of pink spots appears, which spreads from the face and neck to cover the whole body. The disease is mild in effect and generally disappears after a 2-week period. INFECTION with German measles normally confers IMMUNITY. Some women may not be immune because they were either not exposed to the VIRUS or previously vaccinated. If German measles is contracted by a pregnant woman who is not immune, it can cause MISCARRIAGE, STILLBIRTH or serious BIRTH DEFECTS in early PREGNANCY. Hence it is a wise precaution for all women planning to conceive to be tested for ANTIBODIES to the rubella virus and vaccination can be given if necessary. Girls in the UK are routinely vaccinated at age 12–13 so problems and risks are small.

Most people develop antibodies to German measles as they have been exposed at some stage to the virus, which is very common. Birth defects include deafness, CATARACTS, brain damage, heart malformations and abnormal internal organs. An injection of gamma-globulin can help protect a foetus considered to be at risk.

gestation the period during which a fertilized EGG develops into a full-term baby. It averages 266 days from CONCEPTION in humans (280 days from the last menstrual period LMP). Gestation is split into 3 TRIMESTERS according to the physiology of foetal growth.

gland an organ or group of cells that secretes a specific substance or substances. ENDOCRINE GLANDS release substances directly into the BLOOD while exocrine glands secrete onto an epithelial surface via a duct. Some glands produce fluids, e.g. milk from the mammary glands (BREAST), saliva from the sublingual gland, etc. The THYROID GLAND is an endocrine gland releasing HORMONES into the bloodstream. A further system of glands, the lymphatics, occur throughout the body in association with LYMPH vessels.

goitre a disease in which the THYROID GLAND increases in size because of a deficiency of iodine in the diet. The main symptom is swelling of the neck, and it can occur in some AUTOIMMUNE DISEASES such as GRAVE'S DISEASE.

gonads the reproductive organs that produce the GAMETES (sex cells) and some HORMONES. These are the ovaries in women and the testes in men.

GnRH a gonadotropin-releasing HORMONE, produced by the HYPOTHALAMUS. It stimulates the PITUITARY GLAND to produce FSH, LH and PROLACTIN.

gonorrhoea an extremely common venereal or SEXUALLY TRANSMITTED DISEASE that is caused by the bacterium *Neissera gonorrhoeae*. The bacteria are found in the MUCOUS MEMBRANES of the VAGINA, URETHRA, throat and mouth. In 80 per cent of affected women and 20 per cent of affected men no symptoms arise, which makes it more dangerous as irreversible tissue damage can occur before it is diagnosed. If gonorrhoea is not treated it can damage and inflame the FALLOPIAN TUBES and other pelvic organs, and this can arise after only 8–10 weeks. Scar tissue may be produced, increasing the risk of future ECTOPIC PREGNANCY or causing INFERTILITY. Other possible damage includes eye INFECTION that can cause blindness, septicaemia (BLOOD poisoning), gonococcal ARTHRITIS, which may occur in conjunction with a painful skin rash (dermatitis), and INFLAMMATION of heart valves. If a baby is born to a mother with gonorrhoea, it may be infected during passage down the BIRTH CANAL. The baby's eyes are especially vulnerable, and until recently this was a major source of blindness (called opthalmia neonatorum). Symptoms of gonorrhoea include a vaginal discharge (green or yellow-green in colour), DYSURIA, possible inflammation of the RECTUM and a sore throat (in the case of oral sex). To diagnose the disease, swabs of the discharge are obtained and organisms grown and identified in the laboratory. Other samples may be taken from the CERVIX, RECTUM, mouth or throat. PELVIC EXAMINATION may be carried out to ascertain if there is other damage. Treatment is by a single, very large dose of penicillin, or tetracycline if the organism is resistant to penicillin. Follow-up tests are carried out weekly for a month to ensure that the disease has been eradicated, and all sexual contact should be avoided until this is confirmed. Tests for SYPHILIS may be done as gonorrhoea can mask the symptoms of other sexually transmitted diseases.

In PREGNANCY, gonorrhoea can cause MISCARRIAGE or tubal infection in the early months. A vaginal DELIVERY is usually not possible because of the risks to the baby of infection. All sexual partners need to be tested and treated, if necessary, to prevent spread of the infection. It has been known since earliest times (1500 BC) and is a major cause of sterility. (*See also* CONGENITAL INFECTION).

Graafian follicle an ovarian FOLLICLE that develops and matures during each MENSTRUAL CYCLE and that breaks through the OVARY wall to release an EGG (OVULATION). After this process, the Graafian follicle breaks down and forms the CORPUS LUTEUM.

Grave's disease a disorder typified by THYROID GLAND overactivity, enlargement of the gland and protruding eyes. It is caused by ANTIBODY production and is probably an autoimmune response (*see* AUTOIMMUNE DISEASE). Patients commonly exhibit excess METABOLISM (because thyroid HORMONES control this), nervousness, tremor, hyperactivity, rapid heart rate, an intolerance of heat, breathlessness, and so on. Treatment may follow one of three courses: drugs to control the thyroid's production of hormones, surgery to remove part of the gland, or radioactive iodine therapy.

gravid the medical word for pregnant.

gum disease a condition caused by bacteria at the junction between gums and teeth. The bacteria are slow-growing and do not damage the gums until 48 hours after plaque has formed, so careful brushing of teeth to remove plaque can prevent gum disease, which is common in people of all ages and shows as red, inflamed areas that bleed when brushed. If the condition is severe, the gums may retract from the teeth, and these may then become loose or fall out. Flossing between teeth is very important in maintaining the gums in good health. Other gum problems are plaque, mouth ulcers, gingivitis and gumboils. (*See also* DENTAL PROBLEMS).

gynaecological examination a physical check-up paying particular attention to the pelvic organs and BREASTS in order to detect any problems at an early stage and/or to monitor and treat an existing condition. It may be carried out by a family doctor, GYNAECOLOGIST or specialist nurse. A thorough examination includes an internal PELVIC EXAMINATION and discussion of any test results and general health with a doctor. Also, it may involve measurement and recording of height and weight, pulse, temperature and BLOOD PRESSURE. Examination of the mouth, throat, LYMPH glands and THYROID GLAND may be carried out with checks on heart and lungs. The breasts may be inspected for tenderness, lumps, NIPPLE DISCHARGE or skin changes. Laboratory tests may be carried out on URINE samples (for presence of protein, sugar or BLOOD), a CERVICAL SMEAR TEST may be carried out and a BLOOD TEST for ANAEMIA. Other tests may be recommended. (*See also* ANTENATAL CARE; BREAST SELF-EXAMINATION; POSTNATAL CARE).

gynaecologist a doctor or physician who specializes in the study of diseases of women and girls, particularly those relating to the female reproductive system.

H

habitual miscarriage three or more MISCARRIAGES that have happened at the same stage in PREGNANCY, possibly for the same reason. The risk of a fourth pregnancy miscarrying is 25 per cent.

haem a compound containing iron, composed of a pigment that is known as a porphyrin, which confers colour. It combines with a protein called globin in the BLOOD to form HAEMOGLOBIN. The prefix haem- also indicates anything relating to blood.

haematuria the presence of BLOOD in the URINE, which may have come from the kidneys, URETERS, BLADDER or URETHRA. It indicates the presence of INFLAMMATION or disease, such as a stone in the bladder or kidney.

haemoglobin the respiratory substance within RED BLOOD CELLS that contains a pigment responsible for the red colour of BLOOD. It consists of the pigment HAEM and the protein globin and is responsible for the transport of oxygen around the body. Oxygen is picked up in the lungs by arterial blood and transported to the tissues where it is released. This (venous) blood is then returned to the lungs to repeat the process.

haemophilia an hereditary disorder of BLOOD coagulation in which the blood clots very slowly. It is a sex-linked recessive condition carried on the X-CHROMOSOME and hence it affects males, with females being the carriers. There are two types, caused by a deficiency of either one of two coagulation factors in the blood. Haemophilia A is caused by deficiency of factor VIII, and haemophilia B by deficiency of factor IX, called Christmas factor. The severity of the disease depends on how much less of the coagulation factor than normal is present in the blood. The symptoms of haemophilia are prolonged bleeding from wounds and HAEMORRHAGE into joints, muscles and other tissues. In the past, the outlook for haemophiliacs was poor, with few surviving into adult life. Now, however, the condition can be treated by injections or transfusions of plasma containing the missing coagulation factor and, with care, a sufferer can hope to lead a much more normal life.

haemorrhage (bleeding) a flow of BLOOD from a ruptured blood vessel that may occur externally or internally. It is classified according to the type of vessels involved: ARTERY, VEIN or capillary. In addition, a haemorrhage may be primary, i.e. it occurs at the moment of injury. It is classed as reactionary when it occurs within 24 hours of an injury and results from a rise in BLOOD PRESSURE. Thirdly, a secondary haemorrhage occurs after a week or 10 days as a result of INFECTION (sepsis). Haemorrhage from a major artery is the most serious kind as large quantities of blood are quickly lost and death can occur within minutes. Haemorrhages at specific sites within the body are designated by special names, e.g. HAEMATURIA (from the kidney or urinary tract), haemoptysis (from the lungs) and haematemesis (from the stomach).

haemorrhoids (piles) varicose and inflamed VEINS around the lower end of the bowel situated in the wall of the anus. They are classified as internal, external and mixed, depending on whether they appear beyond the anus. They are commonly caused by CONSTIPATION or DIARRHOEA, especially in middle and older age, and may be exacerbated by a sedentary lifestyle. They may also occur as a result of childbearing. Symptoms are bleeding and pain, and treatment is by means of creams, injections and suppositories. Attention to diet (to treat constipation) and regular EXERCISE are important, but in severe cases surgery to remove them may be necessary.

hair loss loss of hair that occurs as a result of several conditions. ALOPECIA is the most common reason, but it can also occur during PREGNANCY or the MENOPAUSE because of fluctuating HORMONE levels. It can be due to hair damage caused by frequent use of harsh chemicals or hot air appliances (e.g. rollers, tongs). It can be an adverse reaction to a prescribed medicine or occur as part of the normal ageing process, STRESS, ANXIETY or illness. Certain skin disorders, e.g. ringworm, can also cause patchy hair loss.

headache pain felt within the head that is thought to be caused by dilation of intracranial arteries or pressure upon them. Common causes are STRESS, tiredness, FEVER accompanying an INFECTION, dyspepsia, high BLOOD PRESSURE, rheumatic diseases and an excess of close work involving the eyes. Headache may indicate the presence of disease or disorder in the brain and also result from injury or concussion. Headaches can also arise as a SIDE-EFFECT of some ORAL CONTRACEPTIVE PILLS. Many drugs are used to treat headaches, and the most common are paracetamol, codeine, aspirin and ibuprofen. (*See also* MIGRAINE.)

heart disease any of many types of disease of the heart, which can be caused by INFECTION, ageing or CONGENITAL DEFECT. The most serious is coronary ARTERY disease, the commonest cause of death in adults. Coronary artery disease is any abnormal condition of the arteries of the heart. The most common form is coronary artherosclerosis (*see* ARTERIOSCLEROSIS). The consequence of this is often a heart attack (coronary thrombosis, myocardial infarction) where a narrowed artery is blocked by a BLOOD CLOT, and the BLOOD flow to part of the heart is restricted. Angina pectoris is commonly present, with symptoms of tightness or dull pain in the chest or severe, choking pain with breathlessness, dizziness and sweating.

The cause of coronary artery disease is not known, but increasing age, OBESITY, DIABETES, smoking, HYPERTENSION and high blood CHOLESTEROL levels are all risk factors. It is particularly related to high consumption of saturated fats and refined carbohydrates in the diet. Lack of EXERCISE and high levels of blood triglycerides are additional risk factors. Women tend to develop heart disease after the MENOPAUSE, and it is often more severe than in men of the same age. Women do not recover as well as men after a heart attack or bypass surgery. Treatment is by drugs, bypass surgery to replace damaged arteries and possibly fitting a pacemaker to correct an irregular heartbeat. Damaged heart valves can also be treated and replaced by surgery.

A healthy diet, plenty of exercise, avoidance of STRESS, losing weight if obese and refraining from smoking can help prevent heart disease.

hepatitis INFLAMMATION of the liver because of the presence of toxic substances or INFECTION caused by VIRUSES. ACUTE hepatitis produces abdominal pain, JAUNDICE, ITCHING, NAUSEA and FEVER. CHRONIC hepatitis has a similar range of symptoms, which may persist for years and lead eventually to cirrhosis. ALCOHOL abuse is a common cause of hepatitis, which may also result as a SIDE-EFFECT of a number of drugs or from overdose. Many virus infections can cause hepatitis, such as HIV and glandular fever. All pregnant women are tested for hepatitis B, as infants born to infected mothers can become chronic carriers. Most contract the virus during DELIVERY, but an injection of the hepatitis B vaccine and gammaglobulin within the first 12 hours of life can give protection. Additional vaccine is given at 1 and 6 months of age.

hereditary disease any disease or disorder that can be transmitted from parents to their offspring.

hermaphrodite a person who has elements of both the male and female sex organs or in whom the sex organs contain both ovarian and testicular cells. This condition is very rare in humans.

hernia the protrusion of a part or whole of an organ out from its normal position within the body cavity. Most commonly, a hernia involves part of the bowel. A congenital hernia is present at birth, a common one being an umbilical hernia, in which abdominal organs protrude into the UMBILICAL CORD. This is caused by a failure during foetal development and can be corrected by surgery. An umbilical hernia can occur in adults, more commonly in women than men. It is caused by a weakness in the abdominal wall and is often associated with previous PREGNANCY and OBESITY. An acquired hernia occurs after birth, a common example being an inguinal hernia, in which part of the bowel bulges through a weak part of the abdominal wall (known as the inguinal canal). Another common type is a hiatus hernia, in which the stomach passes through the hiatus (a hole allowing passage of the oesophagus) from the abdomen into the chest cavity. Strenuous physical activity can lead to the production of a hernia, which usually develops gradually. Although short-term measures are employed to control a hernia or reduce its size, the usual treatment is by means of surgery to return and retain the protrusion in its proper place.

herpes INFLAMMATION of the skin and MUCOUS MEMBRANES characterized by the development of blisters and caused by several types of herpes VIRUS. Herpes simplex I causes COLD SORES of the nose, mouth and face and may be caught in childhood. It recurs from time to time but can be treated with anti-viral agents. Herpes simplex II causes GENITAL HERPES. Other herpes viruses are herpes zoster, which causes chickenpox and shingles, and the Epstein-Barr virus, which causes glandular fever.

heterosexual a sexual relationship between two people of the opposite sex or a person who prefers a sexual partner of the opposite sex.

high-risk pregnancy one that poses a greater than normal risk to the health of the mother and baby. Various CHRONIC diseases, including DIABETES, HYPERTENSION, liver, kidney or HEART DISEASE,

CANCER, SICKLE-CELL ANAEMIA and similar BLOOD disorders, cause higher risks in PREGNANCY. Also, INFECTIONS in the mother, such as GONORRHOEA, SYPHILIS, GERMAN MEASLES, GENITAL HERPES, AIDS, and drug addiction and alcoholism increase the risks. RHESUS INCOMPATIBILITY is now rarely a problem in developed countries. High-risk pregnancies occur in women over 35 or those in their early teens, in MULTIPLE PREGNANCY or where there were previous problems in an earlier DELIVERY. Such women require special ANTENATAL CARE. OBESITY and smoking can lead to PREMATURE or underweight babies and increase the risk of ABRUPTIO PLACENTAE, PLACENTA PRAEVIA or MISCARRIAGE.

hip replacement a surgical operation in which the hip joint is replaced by an artificial ball and socket joint. The operation is done to relieve the CHRONIC PAIN, stiffness and limited movement in a hip affected by OSTEOARTHRITIS with degeneration of the joint or a poorly healed fracture. Hip replacements have a success rate of 90–100 per cent and can allow patients a new lease of life. Repeated hip replacements can be done if problems arise or if the joint wears out. This operation is far more common in women as they are more prone to BONE and joint disorders in later life.

hirsutism excess body and facial hair in women. It can appear as dark hair on the chin, upper lips, around the NIPPLES, on the chest and on the abdomen below the navel. It can be a hereditary trait common in some races. It may be due to excess production of ANDROGENS by the ADRENAL GLANDS or by the ovaries. Hirsutism may be due to CUSHING'S SYNDROME or an adrenal gland tumour. Occasionally it develops as a result of an ENDROCRINE abnormality, causing a virilizing syndrome in which there is AMENORRHOEA, a deep voice and enlarged CLITORIS. Starting or stopping the ORAL CONTRACEPTIVE PILL can trigger excess hair growth, as can PREGNANCY and the MENOPAUSE. Hirsutism can be a symptom of an ovarian tumour or POLYCYSTIC OVARIAN SYNDROME. The excess hair can be removed by shaving, bleaching, depilatories, waxing or electrolysis, but any underlying cause must be investigated and treated.

HIV the human immuno-deficiency VIRUS that causes AIDS.

home birth the DELIVERY of a baby at home, which can be much more relaxed than a HOSPITAL BIRTH. Generally there is no need to travel while in LABOUR, as the woman is attended by a qualified MIDWIFE who remains throughout the labour and birth. Advantages of a home birth include freedom to move around and give birth in any position that is comfortable. The amniotic membranes are allowed to rupture spontaneously, and partner and children can play an integral part in the birth. The labour is controlled by the woman with pain relief available if needed. The baby is born into its own home, and BONDING and BREAST-FEEDING can take place easily. The partner can have a much bigger role in the birth, and the chances of EPISIOTOMY are less than in a hospital delivery. In the event of something going wrong, a hospital delivery may be needed, and this can be discussed beforehand. Home birth requires some preparation and is not suitable in all cases. Women with DIABETES, a MULTIPLE PREGNANCY, complications in previous pregnancies, ANAEMIA, GENITAL HERPES, ECLAMPSIA (or PRE-ECLAMPSIA) or high BLOOD PRESSURE should not plan a home birth. A woman who is past her expected date of delivery or who has a PREMATURE LABOUR should have a hospital birth, as should those with HYDRAMNIOS, ABRUPTIO PLACENTAE, a BREECH presentation, PLACENTA PRAEVIA or a small pelvis. Home births are still in the minority.

homosexual a sexual relationship between two people of the same sex or a person who prefers a sexual partner of the same sex.

hormone a naturally present chemical substance produced by the body that acts as a messenger. A hormone is produced by cells or GLANDS in one part of the body and passes into the bloodstream. When it reaches another specific site, its 'target organ', it causes a reaction there, modifying the structure or function of cells, perhaps by causing the release of another hormone. Hormones are secreted by the ENDOCRINE glands, and examples are the sex hormones, e.g. testosterone, secreted by the testes, and OESTROGEN and PROGESTERONE, secreted by the ovaries.

hormone replacement therapy (HRT) the replacement of the natural HORMONES—OESTROGEN and PROGESTERONE—that are lost after the MENOPAUSE. The menopause can occur in women aged 35 to 60, but most commonly happens between 45 and 55. It can occur following a HYSTERECTOMY, removal of the ovaries and radiation treatment for OVARIAN CANCER. During the menopause levels of oestrogen and progesterone in the body fall, and this can cause HOT FLUSHES, INSOMNIA, DEPRESSION, irritability, night sweats, changes in skin texture, mood swings, VAGINITIS and loss of LIBIDO. The risks of developing OSTEOPOROSIS, HEART DISEASE and STROKE increase significantly after the menopause. Twenty per cent of woman have no obvious symptoms, but the menopause can have a significant adverse effect on women's daily lives.

HRT replaces the hormones that have been lost and alleviates the symptoms of the menopause. Women who still have a UTERUS need progesterone to prevent oestrogen acting alone on the lining of the uterus. Without progesterone there is a slightly higher risk of ENDOMETRIAL CANCER. Women who have had a hysterectomy require only oestrogen. The hormones can be taken in the form of tablets, implants, patches or vaginal creams. A medical examination is carried out prior to being prescribed HRT, and routine checks on BLOOD PRESSURE, BREASTS, and URINE TESTS, etc, are carried out. A regular CERVICAL SMEAR TEST is needed. HRT containing progesterone causes a monthly bleed, and there may be SIDE-EFFECTS such as FLUID RETENTION, bloating, breast tenderness, NAUSEA, HEADACHES, abdominal CRAMPS, dizziness, irritability and irregular bleeding. Changing to another brand of pill with a different balance of hormones can help alleviate some of these, and it may take time to find a formulation that best suits each individual. HRT alleviates many of the symptoms of the menopause and, most importantly, protects against osteoporosis if taken for more than 5 years. Many doctors believe that its role in lessening the impact of osteoporosis (which severely threatens the health and longevity of women) far outweighs any potential risks, although others adopt an opposing view. The therapy should be used for as long as required—some doctors prefer 2, 5 or 10 years, but others recommend HRT for life. HRT carries a slightly increased risk of BREAST CANCER, and it can exacerbate FIBROIDS, ENDOMETRIOSIS, GALLSTONES and GALL BLADDER diseases. However, it may help to protect against heart disease, stroke, ovarian, cervical and endometrial cancer. HRT is not suitable for everyone, and it may not be prescribed for women who smoke, are overweight, have DIABETES, high blood pressure, CHRONIC liver disease or history of thrombosis. Previous history of vaginal, cervical, endometrial or breast CANCER, which are often hormone-dependent, normally rules out HRT. Any abnormal bleeding requires investigation.

hospital birth giving birth in hospital. Some hospitals have BIRTHING ROOMS, which are more like a home environment, less intimidating and more comfortable. This combines the relaxed atmosphere of a HOME BIRTH with the emergency care of a hospital readily available. In hospitals maternity care is controlled by OBSTETRICIANS, doctors, nurses and midwives. In many hospitals women in LABOUR are in the care of a team of midwives (with doctors available if needed). The shaving of PUBIC HAIR, giving enemas and episiotomies used to be carried out routinely in hospital during labour but this is no longer the case, and a woman is now normally consulted prior to any procedure. This also applies to AMNIOTOMY, INDUCTION OF LA-BOUR, use of FORCEPS, FOETAL MONITORING and DELIVERY in a dorsal lithotomy position (flat on back with legs bent). There may still be circumstances (generally in an emergency) in which some of these procedures are needed to accelerate delivery, but they are performed in the best interests of mother and child. Most women are not al-lowed food or drink in labour (because of the risk of sickness if ANAESTHESIA is later needed) but may be given glucose to provide energy if necessary. A woman may be moved into a delivery room or have her movement restricted by foetal monitoring equipment.

The advantages of a hospital birth are to ensure the best out-come for mother and baby, emergency medical assistance is readily available and a special care baby unit is usually on hand if the need arises. Setting out a birth plan to state how the mother would like the labour to be managed can help resolve any possible problems. A birth plan should address the role of the birth partner, pain re-lief, delivery position preferred, type of foetal monitoring and the woman's views on shaving of pubic hair, enema, induction, episi-otomy, amniotomy and the use of drugs These help medical staff, the woman and her partner to work together for a safe birth.

Hospital births are advised in MULTIPLE PREGNANCY, DIABETES, HEART DISEASE, HYDRAMNIOS, BREECH BIRTH, PRE-ECLAMPSIA, ECLAMPSIA, high BLOOD PRESSURE, ANAEMIA, ABRUPTIO PLACENTAE, PLACENTA PRAEVIA, GENITAL HERPES, AIDS, a PREMATURE or late delivery and in mothers with a small pelvis. Some 94 per cent of all deliveries in the UK are in hospital, but many encourage natural childbirth where labour and delivery are controlled by the mother and there is little medical intervention. Active birth enables mothers to be more relaxed, and upright delivery positions usually make labour easier, shorter and lessen the chances of intervention. A partner-assisted birth is common as the partner can help encourage the woman and relieve her pain by massage or other means. Water births are increasing in popularity and can be carried out in hospital or at home. Birthing pools are generally used for pain relief, and such births have less chance of medical intervention. All water births must have a qualified attendant present. (*See also* CAESAREAN SECTION).

hot flushes a sudden sensation of heat that may extend over the whole body or progress up from the chest to the neck and face. They may be followed by sweating and chills. They are the most common symptom of the MENOPAUSE and occur in up to 80 per cent of women. They range in frequency from once a week to 15–20 per day and can be resolved by HORMONE REPLACEMENT THERAPY and may also be helped by supplements of VITAMINS C and E.

human chorionic gonadotropin (HCG) a HORMONE secreted by the PLACENTA during PREGNANCY. HCG maintains the production of PROGESTERONE from the CORPUS LUTEUM, and its presence in the URINE is used as the basis for most pregnancy tests. It may be used to treat female INFERTILITY.

hydatidiform mole an abnormal development of the PLACENTA and the CHORION in which they resemble a bunch of grapes. The EMBRYO dies and disintegrates. The UTERUS is enlarged, and there is vaginal bleeding, severe NAUSEA and VOMITING, and eventually the placental and chorionic tissue are expelled through the VAGINA. It can become apparent in the 3rd or 4th month of PREGNANCY when no foetal heartbeat or movement is detected. ULTRASOUND and exceptionally high levels OF HUMAN CHORIONIC GONADOTROPIN (HCG) in

BLOOD confirm the presence of a hydatidiform mole. Some 80–90 per cent of these growths are BENIGN, but they can become MALIGNANT, giving rise to a CANCER called choriocarcinoma. A D AND C may be required to remove the mole, and levels of HCG need to be checked in the blood until the level has remained negative for one year. After that it is safe to attempt another pregnancy.

hydramnios an excessive amount of amniotic fluid surrounding the FOETUS, often from the 5th month of PREGNANCY. Normally about 1 litre of fluid is present, but more than 2 litres is considered excessive. The increase in amniotic fluid may be gradual or sudden. The symptoms are a swollen UTERUS (which causes breathlessness) and FLUID RETENTION in the legs and abdomen. The condition has no known cause but occurs in MULTIPLE PREGNANCY and in mothers with DIABETES. It is often associated with foetal abnormalities, particularly of the central NERVOUS SYSTEM and gastrointestinal tract. Hydramnios may lead to PREMATURE BIRTH, and there is a foetal death rate of 50 per cent or greater, both before and after birth. The condition is confirmed by ULTRASOUND, and bed rest and sedation can make the mother more comfortable.

hydrosalpinx a condition that often results from INFECTION with GONORRHOEA in which a FALLOPIAN TUBE is filled with fluid and closed at the end nearest the OVARY. This means an egg from that ovary cannot enter the tube, and if the condition appears on both sides (bilaterally) the woman is infertile. This condition can be detected by PELVIC EXAMINATION and confirmed by HYSTEROSALPINGOGRAPHY. An operation called salpingosomy can be carried out to open up the blocked Fallopian tubes.

hygiene the science of maintaining health. Generally associated with applying strict standards of cleanliness, e.g. washing with soap and water, toothbrushing, etc.

hymen a thin membrane that covers the lower end of the VAGINA at birth and usually tears to some extent before a girl reaches PUBERTY.

hypertension or **high blood pressure** BLOOD PRESSURE is measured using a sphygmomanometer and has two components: systolic and diastolic pressure. The systolic is the pressure in the ARTERY that occurs when the left ventricle of the heart contracts. Diastolic pressure is that recorded when the ventricle dilates and refills with BLOOD. A healthy adult has a systolic pressure of 120 mm mercury and diastolic is 80 mm on average (120/80). Primary hypertension is the elevation of systolic and/or diastolic blood pressure on its own. Secondary hypertension occurs because of a disease or condition, e.g. kidney disease. Symptoms of hypertension include HEADACHES, PALPITATIONS, swollen ankles, angina (heart pains) and shortness of breath, but it can be symptomless. Blood pressure rises gradually with increasing age. The artery walls become less elastic, and more pressure is needed to keep the blood flowing. A raised diastolic pressure can damage the heart and blood vessels, and high blood pressure can lead to heart attack, STROKE and CHRONIC disease of the arteries. Untreated hypertension can be very serious. Treatment is weight loss if obese, reduced salt intake, diuretic drugs (to remove salt and water from the blood and lessen its volume) and measures to control STRESS. Drugs such as calcium channel-blockers and beta-blockers are used to treat severe hypertension. Women on the combined ORAL CONTRACEPTIVE PILL may develop hypertension and must then change to the INTRAUTERINE DEVICE or a BARRIER METHOD of CONTRACEPTION. Hypertension can increase risks in PREGNANCY for mother and child, but careful monitoring usually prevents serious problems. Pregnancy can induce hypertension causing PRE-ECLAMPSIA.

hyperthyroidism excessive activity of the THYROID GLAND—an overactive thyroid. It may be caused by increased growth of the gland, by the presence of a tumour or by GRAVE'S DISEASE. Symptoms are weight loss but increased appetite, AMENORRHOEA, DIARRHOEA, trembling hands, heat intolerance and restlessness with quick movements.

hypoglycaemia a condition in which the level of glucose in the BLOOD is too low for normal body functions. It can happen if the blood sugar regulation system is disrupted by starvation, liver disease, pancreatic tumour, severe INFECTION or gastric surgery. It can occur in DIABETES when too much insulin has been used and insufficient carbohydrate eaten. Symptoms include weakness, rapid heartbeat, increased perspiration, tremors and light-headedness. It can lead to coma and convulsions if not treated, and glucose is given either by mouth or injection.

hypomenorrhoea exceedingly light bleeding during the MENSTRUAL CYCLE.

hypophysectomy the surgical removal of the PITUITARY GLAND, occasionally used as part of the treatment for BREAST CANCER.

hypothalamus an area of the forebrain in the floor of the third ventricle, having the thalamus above and PITUITARY GLAND below. It contains centres controlling vital processes, e.g. fat and carbohydrate METABOLISM, thirst and water regulation, hunger and eating, thermal regulation and sexual function. It also plays a part in the emotions and in the regulation of sleep. It controls secretions from the pituitary gland. The hypothalamus produces GNRH, which causes FSH (follicle-stimulating hormone) and LH (luteinizing hormone) production from the pituitary gland.

hysterectomy the surgical removal of the UTERUS (and possibly the ovaries, FALLOPIAN TUBES, CERVIX and top of the VAGINA). It may be performed to treat a life-threatening condition such as invasive CANCER of the reproductive organs, severe uncontrolled bleeding causing ANAEMIA, serious pelvic INFECTION or PROLAPSE of the uterus, and some conditions of the BLADDER or intestines. The operation is also carried out to improve the quality of life for women with severe ENDOMETRIOSIS, FIBROIDS, prolapse, PRECANCEROUS conditions and ADHESIONS. In many cases there are alternatives and hysterectomy is used as a last resort when other treatments fail. There are several types of hysterectomy—subtotal, total (with removal of one or both Fallopian tubes and ovaries) and radical. They may be carried out through an abdominal or vaginal incision or via the cervix. If the ovaries are removed, HORMONE REPLACEMENT THERAPY may be needed. After abdominal surgery, recovery may take up to 3 months, and lifting, overactivity and SEXUAL INTERCOURSE need to be avoided during this time. CERVICAL SMEAR TESTS may still be necessary. Postoperative complications can arise, as with any abdominal surgery, and so a stay in hospital of 8–10 days is likely to be necessary.

hysterosalpingogram an X-RAY picture of the UTERUS and FALLO-

PIAN TUBES that is obtained by injecting a radio-opaque dye. A blockage is easily seen, as are uterine septums in which the womb is an unusual shape. Uterine septums generally restrict the movement of a baby, so normal DELIVERY is not possible. The procedure is not painful and takes about 15 minutes. Hysterosalpinogram is used to investigate INFERTILITY and to examine the site of ECTOPIC PREGNANCY and any damage that may have resulted. This procedure has been replaced to some extent by LAPAROSCOPY.

hysteroscopy the use of a hysteroscope inserted through the CERVIX into the UTERUS to locate and remove an INTRAUTERINE DEVICE. It can also be used in TUBAL LIGATION and removal of FIBROIDS and uterine ADHESIONS.

I

identical twins a MULTIPLE PREGNANCY in which a single fertilized egg divides into two, producing identical individuals of the same sex. It occurs at random in about 1 in every 200 pregnancies.

ileostomy a permanent surgical opening through the abdominal wall in which the ileum or small intestine discharges faeces into a bag. This is performed only when medical treatment has failed to control a condition such as ulcerative colitis. (*See also* COLOSTOMY.)

immune system the BONE MARROW and BLOOD-mediated defence system in vertebrate animals, made up of 4 parts: (1) cell-mediated immune response; (2) humoral (ANTIBODY-mediated) immune response; (3) white blood cells; (4) complement system. This gives both natural and acquired IMMUNITY and stops or limits the growth of pathogens such as VIRUSES, bacteria, etc.

immunity the way in which the body resists INFECTION because of the presence of ANTIBODIES and white BLOOD cells. Antibodies are generated in response to the presence of ANTIGENS of a disease. There are several types of immunity: active immunity is when the body produces antibodies and continues to be able to do so during the course of a disease, whether occurring naturally (also called acquired immunity) or by deliberate stimulation; passive immunity is short-lived and caused by the injection of ready-made antibodies from someone who is already immune.

implantation the attachment of the blastocyst, which has developed from the fertilized EGG, into the wall of the UTERUS. This occurs very early in EMBRYO development, 7 to 10 days after FERTILIZATION. The PLACENTA begins to form after about 12 days, and some women have slight bleeding (implantation bleeding) at this time.

incompetent cervix a rare condition of PREGNANCY in which the CERVIX opens before full term, often in the 3rd or 4th month. The amniotic membranes rupture and a MISCARRIAGE follows. It tends to be a result of injury to the cervix during a previous DELIVERY, D AND C, or other procedure. A woman who was exposed to DES in the WOMB may have this problem, which tends to recur with each pregnancy. Suturing the cervix keeps it closed, and the stitches are normally removed a week before the expected delivery.

incomplete miscarriage a MISCARRIAGE where part of the membranes, FOETUS or PLACENTA is retained. This generally shows as continued bleeding and can be rectified by a D AND C or VACUUM ASPIRATION to remove all material from the UTERUS.

incontinence an inability to control bowel movements or passage of URINE. Urinary incontinence may be caused by a LESION in the brain or spinal cord, injury to the sphincter muscle or damage to the nerves of the BLADDER. STRESS INCONTINENCE is also common in women because of weakening of muscles through childbirth.

incubation period the time between a person being exposed to an infection and the appearance of symptoms. Incubation periods for diseases tend to be quite constant, some commoner ones being measles 10–15 days, German measles 14–21, chicken pox 14–21, mumps 18–21 and whooping cough 7–10 days.

induction of labour stimulating uterine CONTRACTIONS to start LABOUR by artificial means, normally by AMNIOTOMY or using OXYTOCIN. It must be used with caution and for sound medical reasons, as very strong contractions can result in a highly painful labour. If they are too strong they can even rupture the UTERUS, posing a risk to the life of mother and baby. Induction is carried out only if there is significant risk, as in PRE-ECLAMPSIA, HYPERTENSION or if the baby is past its due date and showing signs of distress.

infection the invasion of the body by pathogens, causing disease. Bacteria, VIRUSES, fungi, etc, enter the body and multiply, and after an INCUBATION PERIOD symptoms appear. The organisms reach the body in many ways: as airborne droplets, by direct contact, SEXUAL INTERCOURSE or vectors, or from contaminated food, etc.

infertility the inability to conceive. Subfertility, in which couples have difficulty in conceiving, is quite common (10 per cent of all cases). Female infertility results from three main causes: (1) failure to ovulate is the most common and can be due to damaged ovaries, lack of EGGS or hormonal problems, some of which can be resolved by treatment with fertility drugs; (2) hormonal imbalance after CONCEPTION, which may respond to treatment with drugs; (3) structural problems in which the FALLOPIAN tubes are damaged or blocked (because of pelvic INFECTION or INFLAMMATION, previous surgery, ECTOPIC PREGNANCY or scar tissue) or defect in the UTERUS. The uterus may have a congenital abnormality or be affected by ADHESIONS, FIBROIDS, POLYPS or ENDOMETRIOSIS. The CERVICAL MUCUS may be insufficient or too thick or contain ANTIBODIES that attack the partner's SPERM. These problems are investigated by HORMONE and OVULATION tests, ULTRASOUND scans, BIOPSY of the ENDOMETRIUM, LAPARAROSCOPY or HYSTEROSALPINGOGRAM. Treatment depends on the nature of the problem.

Male infertility results from four main causes: (1) problems with sperm, which are very vulnerable to damage and are affected by influences outside the body. Testicular failure is a rare condition in which semen contains no sperm, and it can result from untreated undescended testicles, chromosomal abnormality (KLINE-FELTER'S SYNDROME), mumps during adult life, or injury. This condition is untreatable but may not affect both testes. Low sperm counts are believed to be becoming increasingly common in young men, and the sperm present may be abnormal. This can be caused by HORMONE, anatomical or immunological problems as well as environmental factors; (2) hormonal problems can arise if the PITUITARY, THYROID or ADRENAL GLANDS are not working properly; (3) anatomical problems can be congenital or develop because of injury, INFECTION or disease. These include hydrocele (excess fluid round the testes) or varicocele (enlarged veins in testes and scrotum), which inhibit sperm production. Also, retrograde ejaculation in which semen travels back to the BLADDER instead of forwards through the URETHRA and blockage of the vas deferens, which connects the testicles to the seminal vesicles; (4) immunological problems can occur if the man's body produces antibodies to his own sperm. These problems can be investigated by sperm, postcoital and egg penetration tests, which assess sperm number, quality, mobility and ability to bring about fertilization.

Around 30 per cent of infertility is due to the male partner, 30 per cent to the female partner, and the rest to problems in both partners. Many can be solved by treatment or methods such as ASSISTED CONCEPTION, e.g. IN VITRO FERTILIZATION, ARTIFICIAL INSEMINATION, etc. (*See also* SIMS-HUHNER TEST.)

inflammation the response of the body's tissues to injury, which involves pain, redness, heat and swelling. The first sign, when the tissues are infected or injured physically or chemically, is a dilation of BLOOD vessels in the affected area, increasing blood flow and resulting in heat and redness. The circulation then slows a little, and white blood cells migrate into the tissues producing the swelling. The white blood cells engulf invading bacteria, dead tissue and foreign particles. After this, either the white blood cells migrate back to the circulation or there is the production and discharge of pus as healing begins. CHRONIC inflammation is when repair is not complete and there is formation of scar tissue.

inflammatory breast cancer a rare CANCER of the breast in which the tumour is very fast-growing and the skin is red, hot and painful. It develops mainly during PREGNANCY and is treated with RADIOTHERAPY and possibly a simple MASTECTOMY operation. CHEMOTHERAPY often follows surgical treatment.

inherited disorder *see* BIRTH DEFECTS.

insemination the injection of semen into the VAGINA.

insomnia the inability to sleep or disturbed sleep patterns. It is a very common problem that can arise because of ANXIETY, STRESS, physical pain, DEPRESSION, the MENOPAUSE, increasing age or jet lag. Insomnia is common during PREGNANCY as urinary frequency increases and also there may be sweating, hot flushes and discomfort from the large bulk of the abdomen. 'Catnapping' during the day is a good way of recovering lost sleep, and sleeping pills should only be used for short periods as they can be addictive. A warm bath or hot drink before bed can help a person to relax and lead to a good night's sleep.

intraductal papilloma an uncommon, wart-like growth in one of the major ducts underneath the NIPPLE and AREOLA. They are more likely to occur in women over 40 and can regress on their own but may cause a discharge from the nipple. On occasions these growths can become MALIGNANT, and hence they are always removed surgically. The condition often recurs.

intrauterine device (IUD) a small device made of plastic or metal that is placed in the UTERUS to prevent PREGNANCY. It is thought to prevent CONCEPTION by interfering with IMPLANTATION of an EMBRYO and possibly making the fluids in the uterus hostile to SPERM. Some IUDs contain copper, which helps to destroy sperm. The IUD must be inserted by a doctor and should be checked every week by the woman (by feeling the threads hanging from it) to make sure it is still in place. Occasionally the IUD is expelled by the uterus, and this is more common in the first few months of use. The IUD is the third most popular form of CONTRACEPTION in the UK (7–8 per cent of women use it), can be used for up to 5 years and has a success rate of 98 per cent. However, it is usually not suitable for women with a previous ECTOPIC PREGNANCY, abnormal uterus, PELVIC INFLAMMATORY DISEASE, GONORRHOEA, FIBROIDS or a history of heavy menstrual bleeding (although a new type available is primarily designed to treat this problem). Also, an IUD may be unsuitable for women with CERVICITIS, ENDOMETRIOSIS, HEART, liver OR SEXUALLY TRANSMITTED DISEASE, DIABETES or ANAEMIA.

An IUD increases the risk of an ectopic pregnancy and pelvic INFECTION, which can lead to INFERTILITY. Also, it may cause heavier periods, CRAMPS and BACK PAIN. If the device is not inserted properly or moves there is a risk that it may perforate the uterus and lodge in the abdomen, which can lead to infection or other serious complications and requires surgical removal. Hence, regular monitoring of the position of the device is vital.

inverted nipple a NIPPLE that is turned inwards instead of protruding outwards. Manipulation of the nipples or wearing a breast shield can encourage the nipple into its normal position, allowing BREAST-FEEDING.

A nipple that becomes inverted after previously being normal may indicate an abnormality, such as a tumour, in the breast. Always see a doctor if you notice any changes in your breasts.

in vitro fertilization (IVF) treatment for INFERTILITY in which mature EGGS are removed from a woman and combined with her partner's SPERM in the laboratory. Any fertilized eggs are examined microscopically and then transferred to her UTERUS, where it is hoped they may implant as normal. The process was developed in the late 1970s and the first 'test-tube baby' was born in 1978. IVF is used for women who have blocked FALLOPIAN TUBES but functional ovaries, or for women with a functional uterus and Fallopian tubes but who do not produce eggs.

A woman is normally given a course of fertility drugs to boost the number of eggs produced, and these are removed by LAPAROSCOPY and cultured with the sperm. A maximum of 3 embryos are inserted into the uterus at any one attempt at PREGNANCY. Any excess embryos may be frozen (for future IVF attempts) or donated to other women (EMBRYO TRANSFER). HORMONES may be given to favour a pregnancy and within 10–16 days it can be determined if the procedure has been successful. Success rates vary between clinics, but generally 45 per cent of women aged up to 34 are pregnant after 6 attempts. After age 34, the chances of pregnancy decline. There are several different techniques used to bring about pregnancy. Gamete intrafallopian transfer (GIFT) transplants sperm and eggs into the Fallopian tubes and allows FERTILIZATION to happen naturally. ZIFT (zygote intrafallopian transfer) is a variation of GIFT in which a ZYGOTE (early embryo) is placed in the Fallopian tube. Tubal embryo stage transfer (TEST) transfers embryos into the Fallopian tube instead of the uterus. POST is peritoneal ovum and sperm transfer, in which sperm and eggs, mixed in a syringe, are injected into the abdomen near the ends of the Fallopian tubes so that they enter the tubes and undergo fertilization as normal. All these variations have been developed with the aim of producing a healthy pregnancy.

irregular periods a MENSTRUAL CYCLE that varies in duration from the usual 28 days and may show no regular pattern. It may result from HORMONE imbalance, STRESS, dieting, ANAEMIA, THYROID GLAND disorder, emotional distress or serious illness including pelvic LESIONS and CANCER. (*See also* BREAKTHROUGH BLEEDING).

itching irritation of the skin that is relieved by scratching. It can be caused by an allergic reaction, dry skin and genital problems. Conditions such as HAEMORRHOIDS, ECZEMA, PUBIC LICE, THRUSH, athlete's foot, ringworm, JAUNDICE, PRURITUS VULVAE, DANDRUFF and GENITAL HERPES can all cause itching. Treatment of each condition is required to stop the irritation.

IUD abbreviation for INTRAUTERINE DEVICE.

J

jaundice a condition characterized by the unusual presence of bile pigment (bilirubin) in the BLOOD. The bile produced in the liver passes into the blood instead of the intestines, and because of this there is a yellowing of the skin and the whites of the eyes. There are several types of jaundice: obstructive, caused by bile not reaching the intestine because of an obstruction, e.g. a GALLSTONE; haemolytic, where red blood cells are destroyed by haemolysis; hepatocellular, caused by a liver disease, such as HEPATITIS, which results in the liver being unable to use the bilirubin. Neonatal jaundice is quite common in newborn infants when the liver is physiologically immature, but it usually lasts only a few days. The infant can be exposed to blue light, which converts bilirubin to biliverdin, another (harmless) bile pigment.

K

Kegel exercises pelvic floor exercises to strengthen the PUBOCOCCYGEOUS muscle. They consist of alternately contracting and relaxing the pubococcygeous muscle, which is the one that controls the flow of URINE. There are three types of exercise that keep the muscles that support the UTERUS, BLADDER and bowel well toned. Tightening and relaxing the muscle 50 times a day is recommended at first and helps to prevent PROLAPSE after DELIVERY and tones up the VAGINA for SEXUAL INTERCOURSE.

Klinefelter's syndrome a genetic disorder in males in which there are 47 rather than 46 CHROMOSOMES, the extra one being an X-CHROMOSOME producing a genetic make-up of XXY instead of the usual XY. The physical manifestations are small testes that atrophy, resulting in a lack of sperm production, enlargement of the BREASTS, long thin legs and little or no facial or body hair. There may be associated mental retardation and pulmonary disease. The disease occurs in 1 in 700 male births and can be detected by AMNIOCENTESIS.

L

labia a pair of tissue folds that protect the vaginal opening. The labia majora are the equivalent of the scrotum in males and extend from the MONS VENERIS to the PERINEUM. The labia minora extend down to the CLITORIS and form a hood around that organ. Both structures have many nerve endings and sebaceous glands, and are exceedingly sensitive.

labour the process of giving birth, from dilation of the CERVIX through to expulsion of the PLACENTA. It usually begins naturally around 280 days after CONCEPTION but may be induced in some circumstances. There are three stages: In the first, uterine CONTRACTIONS begin and the cervix dilates to about 10 cm diameter, allowing passage of the baby's head. The AMNIOTIC SAC usually ruptures at the end of the first stage, but this may occur earlier. Labour differs in every woman each time it takes place—on average it is 12–14 hours for a first baby and 7 hours for subsequent births.

The first stage of labour is split into three phases. The latent phase is the longest (around 8 hours for a first baby); the active phase lasts 3–5 hours and the contractions are stronger and become more painful; the transitional phase is the most intense but lasts for less than an hour. The second stage of labour is the phase when the mother actively pushes the baby out through the BIRTH CANAL. It lasts from full cervical dilation until DELIVERY and may take a maximum of 2 hours in a first labour. The urge to push down is often irresistible, and each contraction moves the baby's head closer to the vaginal opening. Once the head does not slip back between contractions it is said to be 'crowning'. At this stage it is important to let the PERINEUM tissue stretch naturally. The head is usually soon delivered and the baby's nose and air passages will be cleared. After the head is delivered, the rest of the body usually quickly follows with the next contraction. The UMBILICAL CORD is clamped, usually after it stops pulsating, and is cut. As this is happening the baby can be held by the mother. The baby's condition is checked, and he or she is cleaned, weighed and given back to the parents. An APGAR SCORE test is carried out at this time.

In the third stage of labour the UTERUS contracts again to expel the placenta. Putting the baby to the BREAST helps this process. Most hospitals use an intramuscular injection of Syntometrine to promote placental delivery (as it reduces the risk of POSTPARTUM HAEMORRHAGE), and this is normally done moments after the birth of the baby. The placenta is carefully examined to make sure it is intact and no material is retained in the uterus, which could cause a HAEMORRHAGE later on. The area of the VULVA and VAGINA is checked for tears, and any present may be stitched. The last stage of labour may last 10–20 minutes. Massage may help to bring the uterus back to its usual size, and there is a normal vaginal discharge, called LOCHIA, for around 3 weeks after delivery. Some women have AFTERPAINS as the uterus contracts. Any stitches take 5–6 days to dissolve.

The pain of labour can be managed in several ways. Breathing rhythms, different positions, massage, water, ACUPUNCTURE, hypnosis, visualization and vocal sounds all help. The body's natural pain-killers, endorphins, can be stimulated by transcutaneous nerve stimulation (TENS), a Swedish technique. The use of ANALGESIC pain relief is common and includes ANAESTHESIA—local and epidural, sedatives (rarely used) and narcotics. Among those offered are gas and air and Pethidine. The woman's partner, relative or friend can help with many aspects of labour, providing vital encouragement, reassurance and support. (*See also* CAESAREAN SECTION; EFFACEMENT; HOME BIRTH; HOSPITAL BIRTH; NATURAL CHILDBIRTH; PROLONGED LABOUR; VENTOUSE DELIVERY.)

lactation the process of milk secretion by the mammary glands in the BREAST, which begins at the end of PREGNANCY. Colostrum is produced and secreted before the milk. Lactation is controlled by HORMONES and stops when the baby ceases to be breast-fed.

laparoscopy the use of a special instrument called a laparoscope (a type of endoscope) to examine the organs in the abdominal cavity. Carbon dioxide is introduced into the cavity to expand it and make the organs more visible before the laparoscope is inserted. It is used to detect and treat ADHESIONS, blocked FALLOPIAN TUBES, ENDOMETRIOSIS, OVARIAN CYSTS, ECTOPIC PREGNANCY, BIOPSY, STERILIZATION, to remove a stray IUD and for collecting ova for IN VITRO FERTILIZATION. The only discomfort may be chest and shoulder pain caused by residual pockets of gas, which is eventually absorbed and expelled.

laser surgery surgery using a beam of light energy produced by a laser. This is used to treat eye disorders, e.g. short sight, to remove BIRTH MARKS and other abnormal tissue, leaving healthy surrounding tissue intact. It is used to treat ENDOMETRIOSIS, GENITAL HERPES, PRECANCEROUS LESIONS of the CERVIX, VULVA and VAGINA, TUBAL LIGATION and repair of damaged FALLOPIAN TUBES. Laser surgery lessens the risk of INFECTION and reduces the loss of BLOOD and LYMPH because it seals off the vessels.

lesion a wound or injury to body tissues. Also, an area of tissue that, because of damage caused by disease or wounding, does not function fully. Thus, primary lesions include tumours and ulcers, and from them secondary ones may form.

let-down reflex release of milk in the BREASTS, which is triggered by the OXYTOCIN hormone and produced by suckling, a baby's cry or when a feed is due. The hormone forces the milk from the ACINI into the large ducts behind the NIPPLES and is felt as a tightening or tingling sensation. The let-down reflex occurs simultaneously in both breasts and is strongest in the first few weeks of BREAST-FEEDING. Rarely, the reflex fails because of a lack of oxytocin, but this can be given in a nasal spray. (*See also* BREAST-FEEDING; LACTATION.)

leucorrhoea a discharge of white or yellow-coloured mucus from the VAGINA. It may be a normal condition, increasing before and after MENSTRUATION, but a copious vaginal discharge, especially if it has a strong smell, probably indicates an INFECTION in the genital tract. A common cause is THRUSH, but it may also be because of GONORRHOEA or some other SEXUALLY TRANSMITTED DISEASE.

LH (luteinizing hormone) a HORMONE, produced by the PITUITARY GLAND, that is primarily responsible for OVULATION. LH also stimulates production of OESTROGEN and PROGESTERONE (female hormones) from the CORPUS LUTEUM.

libido the desire to participate in sexual activity. It varies in frequency and intensity between people and throughout the lifetime of an individual. Both sexual response and libido are governed by conscious thoughts and feelings, so any changes may be due to psychological or external factors as well as biochemical factors in the body. STRESS, FATIGUE, fear of PREGNANCY, personal problems, illness, some medications and marital conflict can all reduce libido. This may develop into a CHRONIC problem that can be helped by sex therapy.

Pregnancy and MENOPAUSE can result in an increased or decreased libido, depending on the individual. Many women experience a loss or reduction in libido for a time after childbirth, and this is usually attributed to a combination of emotional and hormonal upheaval, tiredness and the demands of a new baby.

life expectancy the length of time a person is expected to live. It differs from country to country, but generally women live longer than men by an average of about 8 years. In the UK in 1900, life expectancy was 49, in 1960 it was 70, and in 1990 it was 79 years.

lightening *see* ENGAGEMENT.

liver spots brown spots on the skin of the hands, face, forearms and other body areas exposed to the sun. They resemble freckles, frequently develop around the MENOPAUSE and are caused by melanin, the pigment that determines skin colour.

LMP (last menstrual period) the first day of the last menstrual period before a PREGNANCY. It is used to calculate the expected DELIVERY date.

lochia discharge from the VAGINA, which occurs after childbirth as the UTERUS heals. It changes in colour from bright red, pink or brown to yellow-white or colourless after about 10 days. It may occur for 14–42 days. Any foul smell indicates INFECTION that requires treatment, usually with antibiotics.

lung cancer growth of MALIGNANT cells in the epithelium of the air passages (bronchi) or lung, which is a very common type of CANCER. It is very hard to detect in the early stages, and symptoms arise only when the disease is quite advanced. Symptoms include recurrent chest problems such as bronchitis or pneumonia, chest pain, persistent cough, loss of weight, breathing difficulties and yellow sputum that may be streaked with blood. The main cause of lung cancer are smoking (80 per cent of all cases) and exposure to industrial air pollution, e.g. asbestos, nickel, chromates, uranium and arsenic. Nonsmokers can inhale other people's smoke (passive smoking), and this can also cause lung cancer. The condition can be detected on a chest X-RAY or fibreoptic bronchoscopy. It is treated with surgery to remove the affected lung tissue, RADIOTHERAPY and CHEMOTHERAPY. The difficulty in detecting the disease means survival rates are poor, and only 13 per cent of all patients live for more than 5 years.

lupus *see* SYSTEMIC LUPUS ERYTHEMATOSUS.

luteinizing hormone *see* LH.

lymph a colourless, watery fluid that surrounds the body tissues and circulates in the LYMPHATIC SYSTEM. It is derived from BLOOD and is similar to plasma, comprising 95 per cent water with protein, sugar, salts and lymphocytes. The lymph is circulated by muscular action, and it passes through lymph nodes that act as filters and is eventually returned to the blood via the thoracic duct (one of the two main vessels of the lymphatic system).

lymphatic system the network of vessels, valves, nodes, etc, that carry LYMPH from the tissues to the bloodstream and help maintain the body's internal fluid environment. Lymph drains into capillaries and larger vessels, passing through nodes and eventually into 2 large vessels (thoracic duct and right lymphatic duct) that return it to the bloodstream by means of the innominate VEINS.

M

malignant a term used in several ways but commonly referring to a tumour that proliferates rapidly, destroys surrounding healthy tissue and can spread via the LYMPHATIC and BLOOD SYSTEM to other parts of the body. The term is also applied to a form of a disease that is more serious than the usual one and is life-threatening, such as malignant smallpox and malignant HYPERTENSION.

mammary duct ectasia a BENIGN condition in which ducts in the BREAST dilate and fill with thick fluid that may be cream, brown or green in colour. The symptoms are NIPPLE DISCHARGE, odd-shaped lumps and pain or a burning sensation in the breast. The severity of the condition varies with age, with women in their twenties experiencing INFLAMMATION and possibly a BREAST ABSCESS. Women in their forties mainly have pain and lumps, and NIPPLE RETRACTION may occur but only in 10 per cent of cases. If the condition is mild it may resolve with antibiotic treatment, but severe cases require the surgical removal of affected ducts.

mammography an X-RAY examination of the BREAST that is used to detect and diagnose breast diseases, especially CANCER. The breasts are compressed between two plates and generally up to 3 pictures are taken. A cancerous area shows as a dense, white patch and can be seen on a mammogram before it can be felt by manual examination.

Mammography can indicate whether a lump is MALIGNANT or BE-
NIGN, and is recommended for all women aged between 50 and 64
once every 3 years. The lowest dose of radiation is used to reduce
exposure. ULTRASOUND and THERMOGRAPHY are other techniques used
to diagnose breast diseases, particularly in women below 50, in whom
tissue is too dense to give clear results with mammography.

mastalgia BREAST pain that may or may not be linked to the MEN-
STRUAL CYCLE. Cyclical mastalgia is linked to a woman's menstrual
cycle and there are symptoms of pain and lumps in both breasts,
possibly with tenderness in the armpits and upper arms. The condition normally worsens before a period and may be severe enough
to disrupt normal life, requiring treatment. Drug treatment is used
only in severe cases, when the problem has been present for more
than 6 months, but changes in diet may benefit some women. Con-
suming less saturated fat, more gamma-linolenic acid (GLA) and/
or fish oils may help to reduce breast tenderness and resolve mild
mastalgia. The condition is not caused by FLUID RETENTION so diuretic drugs do not help. Mastalgia appears to result from sensitivity to OESTROGEN and PROGESTERONE (female HORMONES), which may
be connected to low levels of GLA in the body. Saturated fats increase the effects of these hormones on the breast and so exacerbate the problem.

The other form is non-cyclical mastalgia, and it is not linked to
the menstrual cycle. There is burning or stabbing breast pain, often
only on one side, which can be constant or occasional. This is a
symptom of such conditions as BREAST CYSTS, INTRADUCTAL PAPIL-
LOMA, MAMMARY DUCT ECTASIA and SCLEROSING ADENOSIS. This type
of breast pain can also result from muscular or skeletal problems,
shingles, BREAST CANCER or a condition called Tietze's syndrome,
which affects the ribs. Treatment is the same as in cyclical mastalgia, and wearing a good supporting bra is important.

mastectomy the partial or complete surgical removal of the BREAST,
normally carried out as a treatment for BREAST CANCER. There are
several different kinds of mastectomy operation, depending on the
amount of tissue removed. With lumpectomy, or partial mastectomy, the tumour and possibly some surrounding tissue is removed,

which has some effect on breast shape. The more radical types of mastectomy are done only as a last resort to save life as they are mutilating and often include removal of the LYMPH nodes in the armpit and the pectoral muscles. A simple or modified radical mastectomy is the most common and removes only the breast tissue and possibly one lymph node to check for spread of the cancer. Normally a BIOPSY is first performed on the lump to determine if it is cancerous and the stage of the disease.

After mastectomy, recovery can be difficult. The scars may not heal for about 2 weeks, and the adjacent arm can often be swollen with restricted movement. There may be significant emotional problems in adjusting to the loss, which require support and reassurance from family and medical staff. Many women need CHEMO-THERAPY and/or RADIOTHERAPY and check-ups at three-monthly intervals. A breast prosthesis can be fitted to restore normal shape, or reconstruction surgery may be carried out at a later date (*see* BREAST PLASTIC SURGERY). Certain charities and self-help groups give advice and help regarding mastectomy and its effects.

mastitis inflammation of the BREAST, usually because of bacterial INFECTION during BREAST-FEEDING. Symptoms include pain in the affected breast, tenderness, swelling, FEVER and possibly a chill. Treatment with warm compresses and antibiotics normally resolves the condition. If the inflammation does not subside then a BREAST ABSCESS may form.

masturbation physical self-stimulation of the external genital organs in order to produce sexual pleasure and possibly ORGASM. Masturbation is considered a normal part of ADOLESCENCE and PUBERTY and is not harmful in any way.

measles an extremely infectious disease, common in childhood, that is caused by a VIRUS. It causes a high FEVER, cough, sneezing and a characteristic rash. It is not usually serious but complications can arise, including pneumonia and middle ear INFECTIONS (which can lead to deafness) and occasionally death. A vaccine is available and has reduced the incidence of measles. Most infants in the UK are immunized against measles with combined MMR vaccine (measles, mumps and rubella).

meconium the first stools of a newborn baby, usually a blackish, dark green in colour. It is made up of bile pigments, mucus and cell debris swallowed by the baby while still in the WOMB. The presence of meconium in the amniotic fluid is a sign of foetal distress because of lack of oxygen. In a BREECH BIRTH, meconium is normally expelled into the VAGINA during LABOUR. After birth, once feeding has started, the meconium is replaced by faeces.

menarche the start of MENSTRUATION for the first time, which occurs between 9 and 18 years of age. Menarche generally takes place 3 or 4 years after the first signs of PUBERTY and is related to the CRITICAL WEIGHT of young girls. Menarche before 9 may be PRECOCIOUS PUBERTY or because of a disease affecting the ENDOCRINE organs. At first, the menstrual periods may be irregular, vary in amount of bleeding and are normally ANOVULATORY (no eggs released). They usually settle down into a regular pattern after a period of time.

menopause (change of life, climacteric) the period before and including the end of MENSTRUATION. This normally occurs between the age of 45 and 55, but a premature menopause may happen earlier, before the age of 40. The ovaries stop producing EGGS, MENSTRUAL FLOW ceases, and the woman is no longer able to have children. Generally, the menopause arises gradually, with menstrual periods changing in frequency and level of flow. After periods have ceased for 12 months, the menopause is usually complete and the woman is said to be postmenopausal. There is a hormonal imbalance in the body during the menopause, with less OESTROGEN from the ovaries and a higher level of FSH (follicle-stimulating hormone) to compensate. This causes menstrual irregularities and other symptoms. Physical symptoms include HOT FLUSHES, night sweats and FATIGUE, and there may be VAGINITIS, PAINFUL INTERCOURSE and VAGINAL ATROPHY. Postmenopausal women run an increased risk of OSTEOPOROSIS. The hormone imbalance can also cause ANXIETY, DEPRESSION, emotional problems, irritability, INSOMNIA and tearfulness. Many of these symptoms can be resolved by HORMONE REPLACEMENT THERAPY, which is becoming increasingly popular. BIRTH CONTROL is necessary until periods have stopped for a year, and regular physical examinations should be carried out, e.g. BLOOD PRESSURE, weight, breasts, pelvic organs and a CERVICAL SMEAR TEST. BREAST SELF-EXAMINATION is important. Any bleeding after the menopause should be investigated to eliminate the possibility of CANCER. The menopause can occur after surgery to remove the ovaries, and in this case it may occupy a short time period and problems can be more severe. (*See also* VAGINITIS; MENSTRUAL CYCLE).

menorrhagia MENSTRUATION with abnormally heavy or prologed blood flow. This may be frequent periods (every 21 days or less), one that continues for 7 days or more, or one with exceptionally heavy flow over 2–3 days. Menorrhagia can occur because of FI-BROIDS, INFLAMMATION in the pelvic cavity, an INTRAUTERINE DEVICE (IUD) or hormonal imbalance. The bleeding can cause ANAEMIA with pallor and fatigue, which can be treated with iron supplements. Treatment depends on the cause and may include a D AND C, the combined contraceptive pill, removal of an IUD, or danazol, a drug that inhibits the HORMONES produced by the PITUITARY GLAND. (*See also* ENDOMETRIOSIS.)

menstrual cup a plastic device shaped like a bell used to collect MENSTRUAL FLOW. It is inserted just inside the VAGINA and can be re-used many times. It is particularly popular in America.

menstrual cycle the periodic sequence of events that prepares the lining of the UTERUS for IMPLANTATION of a fertilized EGG and normally ends in MENSTRUATION. The cycle can vary between 23–25 days, but the average length is 28 days. The menstrual cycle is regulated by the interaction and levels of certain HORMONES that control maturation and release of an egg from the OVARY, development of the ENDOMETRIUM and shedding of this as blood when no PREGNANCY occurs.

The cycle begins on the first day of MENSTRUAL FLOW when the endometrium starts to be shed. This results from decreasing levels of OESTROGEN and PROGESTERONE, which stimulate the HYPOTHALAMUS to produce GnRH (gonadotropin-releasing hormone). This acts on the PITUITARY GLAND and starts secretion of FSH (follicle-stimulating hormone) and LH (luteinizing hormone). FSH stimulates several follicles in the ovary to grow, while LH starts the production of OESTROGEN by the ovarian follicles. This is the proliferative phase of the menstrual cycle, which lasts until OVULATION. At this time all but one of the ovarian follicles die, and the remaining GRAAFIAN FOLLICLE continues to develop while the endometrium in the womb thickens to receive a fertilized egg. High oestrogen levels restrict the amount of FSH, but LH remains constant. In the middle of the cycle, the pituitary is stimulated to produce a large quantity of LH, causing the Graafian follicle to mature, release an egg and degenerate to form the CORPUS LUTEUM, which produces oestrogen and PROGESTERONE.

This signals the end of the proliferative stage and the start of the secretory phase, in which progesterone is predominant. The endometrium continues to thicken, and the uterine glands produce substances that will support a fertilized egg. If FERTILIZATION occurs, the corpus luteum is controlled by HUMAN CHORIONIC GONADOTROPIN (HCG) produced by the developing PLACENTA. If the egg is not fertilized, LH and FSH levels fall in response to increased oestrogen and progesterone production by the corpus luteum. The decline in LH causes the corpus luteum to degenerate and stop producing hormones. Thus the endometrium is not maintained and is shed as blood (and CERVICAL MUCUS) in the menstrual flow. The cycle is then repeated.

menstrual extraction a method of removing menstrual fluids using suction or aspiration so that there is no MENSTRUAL FLOW. A syringe is inserted through the CERVIX at the beginning of the menstrual period and the menstrual fluid is sucked out under negative pressure. It is used as a method of postcoital ABORTION before a PREGNANCY can be confirmed. It may be done within a week of MENSTRUATION, and some people consider it the same as VACUUM EXTRACTION methods of abortion. The procedure has associated risks of damage to the VAGINA or UTERUS, which can lead to INFECTION or PELVIC INFLAMMATORY DISEASE. The technique is not popular in Europe but is used in the USA.

menstrual flow vaginal bleeding that happens as a result of the MENSTRUAL CYCLE. The bleeding normally lasts 2–7 days and is called the **menstrual period**. The fluid consists mainly of BLOOD but also CERVICAL MUCUS, bacteria and cells from the ENDOMETRIUM. The normal pattern of flow differs from woman to woman, both in amount and number of days. It also varies throughout the lifetime of an individual. The main methods of dealing with it are sanitary pads and tampons. Other methods include MENSTRUAL EXTRACTION, MENSTRUAL CUP or MENSTRUAL SPONGE. (*See also* BREAKTHROUGH BLEEDING; DYSMENORRHOEA; HYPOMENORRHOEA; MENORRHAGIA; OLIGOMENORRHOEA; POLYMENORRHOEA.)

menstrual sponge a small natural sponge that is inserted into the VAGINA to soak up MENSTRUAL FLOW, in a similar way to a tampon.

menstruation the monthly discharge of blood, cervical mucus, bacteria and cells from the uterus of non-pregnant women, which occurs between puberty and the menopause (*see* MENSTRUAL CYCLE; MENSTRUAL FLOW).

metabolism the sum of all the physical and chemical changes within cells and tissues that maintain life and growth. The breakdown processes that occur are known as catabolic (catabolism), and those that build materials up are called anabolic (anabolism). The term may also be applied to describe one particular set of changes, e.g. protein metabolism.

metastasis the process by which a MALIGNANT tumour spreads to a distant part of the body, and also the secondary growth that results from this. The spread is accomplished by means of three routes, the BLOOD circulation, LYMPHATIC SYSTEM and across body cavities.

midwife a person other than a doctor who is a specialist in childbirth and qualified to care for a woman before, during and after LABOUR and DELIVERY. The role of a midwife depends on whether the person works in a hospital, community setting or in a domino scheme. The 'domino midwife' comes to the woman's home when labour starts, accompanies her to hospital and delivers the baby. Other midwives provide continuous care throughout PREGNANCY and delivery. Hospital midwives have a variety of different roles, sometimes working as members of a team headed by either an OBSTETRICIAN or senior midwife. (*See also* HOME BIRTH; HOSPITAL BIRTH; OBSTETRICIAN.)

migraine a very severe throbbing HEADACHE, usually on one side of the head, that is often accompanied by disturbances in vision, NAU-

SEA and VOMITING. Migraine is a common condition and seems to
be triggered by any one or several of various factors. These include
ANXIETY, FATIGUE, watching television or video screens, loud noises,
flickering lights (e.g. strobe lights), and certain foods such as cheese
and chocolate or alcoholic drinks. The cause is uncertain but may
involve constriction followed by dilation of BLOOD vessels in the
brain and an outpouring of fluid into surrounding tissues or a disturbance of the balance of serotonin, a neurotransmitter. Attacks
range in severity and can last for several days or even weeks (in
very rare cases). Treatment is by means of pain-relieving drugs such
as aspirin, bed rest in a quiet, dark room, and sleep. Some people
have frequent severe migraines and are treated with PROPHYLACTIC
drugs to stop them developing. These include beta-blockers,
pizotifen and imigran.

mini-pill a name commonly given to the PROGESTERONE-only contraceptive pill. It can prevent OVULATION in some women but also changes
the CERVICAL MUCUS and makes it inhospitable to SPERM. The mini-
pill does not produce any of the SIDE-EFFECTS associated with the
combined ORAL CONTRACEPTIVE PILL. It can give rise to irregular MEN-
STRUAL CYCLES, no periods at all in some women, or BREAKTHROUGH
BLEEDING. The mini-pill has a success rate of 92– 98 per cent, and
many women combine its use with a method of barrier CONTRACEP-
TION such as the DIAPHRAGM or CONDOM. The progesterone-only pill
can be used by women for whom the combined contraceptive pill is
contraindicated and can be used during BREAST-FEEDING. Many
women find this preparation helpful in regulating periods, and it can
lessen the impact of period pains and PREMENSTRUAL TENSION.

Possible side-effects include irregular bleeding, HEADACHES, weight
gain, loss of LIBIDO, hair growth and an increased risk of OVARIAN
CYSTS or ECTOPIC PREGNANCY. The effectiveness of the pill falls if the
woman weighs more than 11 stone (70 kg). The main drawback
with the progesterone-only pill is that no more than 27 hours must
pass between pills for the method to be effective. This means a set
time should be established to take the medication. If a pill is taken
late or missed, another method of contraception needs to be used
for 7 days until the hormonal balance returns.

miscarriage (spontaneous or natural ABORTION) the loss of a FOETUS before the 28th week of PREGNANCY. After 28 weeks, death of the foetus is known as a STILLBIRTH. The spontaneous abortion of a foetus is probably even more common than figures show, as many pregnancies miscarry before they are known. A third of all first pregnancies miscarry, possibly because of an immature UTERUS or genetic or physical defects in the foetus. Some 15–20 per cent of all CONCEPTIONS end in miscarriage, the majority in the first three months of pregnancy.

A miscarriage can occur because of maternal or foetal factors, including defects of the EGG or SPERM, uterine FIBROIDS, hormonal deficiency (too little PROGESTERONE), defects in the anatomy of the uterus, INCOMPETENT CERVIX, severe high BLOOD PRESSURE, RHESUS INCOMPATIBILITY, maternal INFECTION of the reproductive organs, e.g. SYPHILIS and GENITAL HERPES, placental insufficiency, uterine scar tissue and ENDOMETRIOSIS. The risk of a miscarriage increases with a woman's age. Also exposure to certain industrial chemicals, radiation, tobacco smoke and consumption of certain foods or drinks (ALCOHOL) may contribute to miscarriage. The reasons can be investigated through tests, including X-RAY of the uterus, endometrial BIOPSY, BLOOD tests for hormone and ANTIBODY levels, CHROMOSOME and semen analysis.

The main symptoms of a miscarriage are bleeding from the VAGINA, backache and abdominal CRAMPS. Not all miscarriages are the same, and doctors generally define 6 different types. Threatened miscarriage does not necessarily lead to the loss of the foetus. Often the CERVIX remains closed as the abdominal cramps are not strong enough to cause dilation. If it happens early in pregnancy, the miscarriage is normally caused by defects in the foetus, and in this case medical intervention is to little avail. Later in pregnancy, bed rest and drugs to relax the uterus may prevent a threatened miscarriage and delay birth until the foetus is more mature. Miscarriage is inevitable when there is severe bleeding and/or cramps at any stage in pregnancy. No medical treatment can help, as the cervix is usually dilated and the AMNIOTIC SAC has ruptured. An incomplete miscarriage is one in which not all the membranes, foetus and PLACENTA are expelled. This results in continued vaginal bleeding so that a D AND C or VACUUM ASPIRATION needs to be carried out to remove all the material from the uterus. A missed miscarriage is when the foetus dies inside the uterus and remains there. This is more difficult to detect as the symptoms are more vague. There may be vaginal bleeding, reduction in breast size and the uterus stops growing. Some women feel depressed, with FATIGUE or lassitude. Normally contractions begin spontaneously and the foetus is expelled. Otherwise foetal death is eventually detected during ANTENATAL CARE, and the woman has to have a D and C or INDUCTION OF LABOUR by OXYTOCIN. A septic miscarriage is one in which the uterus becomes infected, and this may occur if the foetus has died and started to deteriorate. The symptoms include tenderness of the uterus and abdomen, FEVER, chills and vaginal bleeding. Large doses of antibiotics are needed to treat the infection. HABITUAL MISCARRIAGE is when a woman loses a foetus at the same stage in pregnancy 3 or more times.

Miscarriage can be a deeply distressing occurrence, with feelings of guilt, anger, fear and grief. Reassurance and counselling are important, and a period of mourning is often experienced. A self-help group now exists to provide comfort and support. It may also help to know that many parents go on to have a healthy child from a subsequent preganancy. (*See also* ABORTION.)

mittelschmerz cramping pain in the lower abdomen, which some women experience midway between menstrual cycles around the time of OVULATION. The pain can be quite severe, and there may be some degree of vaginal bleeding.

mole a dark-coloured pigmented spot in the skin that is usually brown. It may be flat or raised and have hair protruding from it. Some types can turn MALIGNANT. (*See also* SKIN CANCER.)

monozygotic twins IDENTICAL TWINS who are derived from a single fertilized egg. (*See also* MULTIPLE PREGNANCY.)

mons veneris the mount of fatty tissue that lies over the central portion of the pubic BONE. After PUBERTY it becomes covered in PUBIC HAIR, forming a triangular pattern called the escutcheon.

mood changes mood changes are a natural response to everyday life. At certain times in life, mood changes can be out of character for a person and may result from illness or HORMONE imbalance. Moodiness and DEPRESSION can occur during PREGNANCY, as part of PREMENSTRUAL TENSION, at the onset of the MENOPAUSE, after childbirth if POSTNATAL DEPRESSION develops, or be due to ANXIETY. Treatment may be necessary, depending on the cause, but usually people cope with occasional changes in mood, and adverse feelings pass.

morning-after pill *see* EMERGENCY CONTRACEPTION.

morning sickness a popular name for the NAUSEA that often occurs in early PREGNANCY—*nausea gravidarum*. It generally occurs in the first three months and then declines, but it can affect some women continually until DELIVERY. The cause is not precisely determined, but it appears that increasing HORMONE levels may irritate the stomach lining, and low BLOOD sugar may contribute. Nausea can be prompted by the smell of tobacco smoke or cooking. The main symptoms are feelings of nausea, retching, VOMITING and an intolerance of some foods, e.g. protein-rich ones such as meat. The main remedy is to prevent low blood sugar by eating small snacks throughout the day, avoiding fatty foods and coffee and having a biscuit or dry toast before rising from bed. Drinking extra fluids helps prevent dehydration if vomiting is occuring. In severe cases, a condition called *hypermesis gravidarum* develops in which frequent vomiting depletes the mother of fluid and minerals. This requires hospitalization so that fluids can be given intravenously. Changing eating habits normally helps to resolve the problem. Anti-nausea medication should be avoided and only ever taken under medical supervision.

mucous membrane a glandular membrane lining nearly all body cavities that have an external opening, e.g. mouth, nose, RECTUM and VAGINA. It secretes mucus that lubricates the tissues it lines.

mucus plug a small pad of mucus that blocks the cervical canal during PREGNANCY. It is usually expelled spontaneously in a fluid discharge with some BLOOD (called 'bloody show') as the cervix slowly dilates. This may occur during the last weeks of pregnancy but usually happens just prior to or during LABOUR.

multigravida a woman who has been pregnant more than once.

multipara a woman who has delivered more than one viable infant.

multiple pregnancy PREGNANCY in which there is more than one
FOETUS—the most common being twins but triplets, quadruplets
and quintuplets can also occur. There are two basic types of multiple pregnancy—monozygotic or identical, in which a single EGG
splits into two or more individuals, and dizygotic or fraternal, where
two or more eggs are fertilized during the same MENSTRUAL CYCLE.
Monozygotic babies develop from a single sperm and egg, while
dizygotic babies involve two or more eggs and sperm. The Dionne
quintuplets, born in Canada in 1934, were the first known set of
monozygotic quins to survive. Identical twins are the same sex and
closely resemble each other, while fraternal twins do not. Identical
twins arise entirely by chance and occur in 1 in every 200 pregnancies. Fraternal twins occur if there are high levels of FSH (follicle-
stimulating hormone) and are more common in black women. They
also occur if there is a family history of twins as polyovulation
(producing more than one egg at OVULATION) is an hereditary trait.
The chance of having fraternal twins increases with age and the
number of previous pregnancies a woman has had.

A multiple pregnancy is suspected if a woman is larger than her
dates suggest, if there is a raised ALPHA-FETOPROTEIN level at week
18. The condition can be detected through ULTRASOUND scans and
listening to foetal heartbeat. Multiple pregnancy increases the
amount of iron and folic acid required and puts more strain on the
mother's body. Increased BLOOD PRESSURE and bodyweight are more
likely to be a problem, and diet requires careful attention. Adequate
rest helps the body to cope with the extra demands. In some cases,
a multiple pregnancy is not suspected until the birth takes place.
The risks to mother and babies are higher in multiple pregnancy,
with a greater rate of MISCARRIAGE and STILLBIRTH. Twins normally
have a shorter GESTATION period and are delivered around 37 weeks
on average. They have a lower BIRTH WEIGHT, and the second baby
to be delivered is at greater risk as it has to withstand more contractions. A multiple labour is usually longer than normal and is
best managed in hospital as one or more of the babies may need to
be delivered by CAESAREAN SECTION. Some conditions such as

HYDRAMNIOS, PROLONGED LABOUR, PRE-ECLAMPSIA, POSTPARTUM HAEM-
ORRHAGE, PLACENTA PRAEVIA and ABNORMAL PRESENTATION are more
common in multiple births. Mortality both before and after birth is
4 times higher than in single births. (*See also* SUPERFECUNDATION;
SUPERFETATION.)

multiple sclerosis (MS) a disease of the brain and spinal cord that
affects the myelin sheaths of nerves and disrupts their function. It
usually affects people below the age of 40, and its cause is unknown
but is the subject of much research. The disease is characterized by
the presence of patches of hardened (sclerotic) connective tissue irregularly scattered through the brain and spinal cord. At first the
fatty part of the nerve sheaths breaks down and is absorbed, leaving
bare nerve fibres, and then connective tissue is laid down. Symptoms
depend on the site of the patches in the central NERVOUS SYSTEM, and
the disease is characterized by periods of progression and REMISSION.
However, they include unsteady gait and apparent clumsiness, tremor
of the limbs, involuntary eye movements, speech disorders, BLADDER
dysfunction and paralysis. The disease can progress very slowly, but
generally there is a tendency for the paralysis to become more marked.
In women, MENSTRUATION and FERTILITY are not affected. The modern view is that PREGNANCY, LABOUR and DELIVERY are not affected by
MS and that the risks of the disease being exacerbated by birth are
only slightly increased. With careful monitoring there should be a
healthy outcome for both mother and baby.

muscular dystrophy any of a group of diseases that involve wasting of muscles and in which an hereditary factor is involved. The
disease is classified according to the groups of muscles that it affects and the age of the person. It usually appears in childhood and
causes muscle fibres to degenerate and to be replaced by fatty and
fibrous tissue. The affected muscles eventually lose all power of
contraction, causing great disability, and affected children are prone
to chest and other INFECTIONS that may prove fatal in their weakened state. The cause of the disease is not entirely understood, but
the commonest form, Duchenne muscular dystrophy, is sex-linked
and recessive. Hence, it nearly always affects boys, with the mother
as a carrier, and appears in very early childhood.

myalgic encephalomyelitis (ME) a disorder in which there is muscular pain, FATIGUE, general DEPRESSION, loss of concentration and
memory, and possibly blurred vision. The cause of the disease is
not understood, but 80 per cent of cases seem to result from viral
infections such as enteroviruses (HEPATITIS and gastric 'flu) or HER-
PES (e.g. glandular fever and chickenpox). The disease tends to be
CHRONIC, and only 20–35 per cent of people recover within 2 years.
The disease tends to develop in the 20–40 age group, and the majority of sufferers are women. The treatment recommended is plenty
of rest and gradual return to exercise. Some people find magne-
sium, gamma-linolenic acid, VITAMIN and mineral supplements help,
as can special diets and homoeopathy.

myasthenia gravis a serious and CHRONIC condition of uncertain
cause, which may be an AUTOIMMUNE DISEASE. It is more common
among young people, especially women (men tend to be affected
over the age of 40). Rest and avoidance of unnecessary exertion is
essential to conserve muscle strength as there is a reduction in the
ability of the neurotransmitter acetylcholine to effect muscle contraction. There is a weakening that affects skeletal muscles and those
for breathing and swallowing, etc. However, there is little wasting
of the muscles themselves. It seems the body produces ANTIBODIES
that interfere with the acetylcholine receptors in the muscle, and
that the thymus GLAND may be the original source of these receptors.
Surgical removal of the thymus gland is one treatment that may be
carried out.

N

natural childbirth *see* PREPARED CHILDBIRTH.
natural family planning a method of CONTRACEPTION and PREGNANCY
planning that is based on timing SEXUAL INTERCOURSE so as to avoid
(or determine) a woman's fertile period (around OVULATION). There
are 4 main ways of calculating ovulation—calendar method, temperature method, CERVICAL MUCUS method, and the combined or

sympto-thermic method. The calendar method requires a woman to record her MENSTRUAL CYCLE for at least 6 months. Then the information about previous menstrual cycles is used to calculate the probable time of ovulation and the fertile period by subtracting 18 from the shortest cycle and 11 from the longest one. Thus, to reduce the chance of pregnancy, vaginal intercourse must be avoided from the first to the last fertile day. This is the least reliable method of natural family planning and does not work in women with IR-REGULAR PERIODS or after childbirth.

The temperature method uses a record of a woman's BASAL BODY TEMPERATURE to determine ovulation. PROGESTERONE released by the CORPUS LUTEUM after ovulation causes a rise in temperature of at least 0.2° C, which can be detected. Over a period of 6–8 months, this can give an idea of a woman's pattern of ovulation. The cervical mucus method involves examining this secretion each night to monitor its quantity and consistency. At ovulation the mucus becomes clear, slippery and often more profuse, and may be apparent externally. The sympto-thermic method combines the temperature and cervical mucus method to estimate the fertile period and is the most reliable. The advantages of natural family planning are that it does not harm the body and gives a woman a better understanding of the working of her body and menstrual cycle. The methods require little equipment, have no SIDE-EFFECTS and are easily reversible. The disadvantages are that they require commitment, patience and self-control in both partners, and a woman may need some initial instruction in how to record the changes. These methods are not completely reliable and inhibit spontaneity, in that sexual intercourse must be avoided for quite long periods of time. They work best for those in a committed and caring relationship where both partners are prepared to overcome any difficulties.

nausea a feeling of being about to vomit. It may be caused by motion sickness, pain, food poisoning, MORNING SICKNESS, drugs, MIGRAINE, HYPOGLYCAEMIA, JAUNDICE and gastric problems.

neonatal a term that relates to the first 28 days of life.

nervous system the complete system of tissues and cells responsible for conducting electrical impulses through the body. It includes nerves, neurones, synapses and receptors (special cells sensitive to a particular stimulus). The nervous system operates through the transmission of impulses that are conducted rapidly to and from muscles, organs, etc. It consists of the central nervous system (brain and spinal cord) and the peripheral nervous system that includes the cranial and spinal nerves.

neural tube defects a class of serious BIRTH DEFECTS in which a baby's spinal cord fails to close properly during development in the womb. If the spinal cord does not close at the top, the brain fails to develop properly (anencephaly) and the baby dies a few hours after birth. If the problem arises lower down, the condition is called SPINA BIFIDA.

nipple a protruding nodule on the BREAST, in females being the area from which milk is expressed during LACTATION. The nipple is usually cylindrical and a brownish colour, darker than the AREOLA. In some women the nipple may be level with the areola or turned inward (inverted). This is not a problem unless a woman wishes to breast-feed. Wearing a breast shield can encourage the nipple to protrude. The nipple contains muscle fibres that make it stand erect if stimulated by cold or sexual excitement. The terminal milk ducts of each breast pass through the nipple.

nipple discharge discharge from the nipple (other than milk) that can indicate disease, disorder or INFECTION. Discharge may be caused by some TRANQUILLIZERS, infection such as MASTITIS, an ENDOCRINE disorder of the PITUITARY GLAND or HYPOTHALAMUS or BENIGN or MALIGNANT TUMOURS, especially INTRADUCTAL PAPILLOMA and PAGET'S DISEASE OF THE NIPPLE. (*See also* BREAST-FEEDING; BREAST SELF-EXAMINATION; LACTATION.)

nipple retraction a condition in which the NIPPLE is pulled inward by an underlying tumour or INFLAMMATION in the breast. Any ulceration, scaling or reddening of the nipple can also indicate disease. (*See also* BREAST CANCER.)

nucleic acid a linear molecule that occurs in two forms: DNA (deoxyribonucleic acid) and RNA (ribonucleic acid), composed of 4 NUCLEOTIDES. DNA is the major part of CHROMOSOMES in the cell nucleus while RNA is found outside the nucleus and is involved in protein synthesis.

nucleotide the basic molecular building block of the NUCLEIC ACIDS RNA and DNA. A nucleotide comprises a 5-carbon sugar molecule with a phosphate group and an organic base. The organic base can be a purine, e.g. adenine and guanine, or a pyrimidine, e.g. cytosine and thymine as in DNA. In RNA uracil replaces thymine.

nullipara a woman who has never given birth to a viable baby.

nurse a person who is trained and experienced in medical knowledge and entrusted with caring for the sick or infirm.

nutrition (nourishment) for a healthy diet, it is important to consume a balance of carbohydrates, proteins, fats, fibre, vegetables and fruit. Carbohydrates are starches and sugars, and they are the body's main source of energy. Health authorities now recommend that people should eat more starchy foods like potatoes, bread, rice, maize and pasta, and reduce sugar intake, particularly of the type found in cakes, biscuits, chocolate, etc. Proteins are required for growth and repair of body cells, and on digestion, are broken down into their constituent amino acids. These are used to form new proteins inside cells. Humans require 8 essential amino acids from food as these cannot be produced in the body. They include valine, leucine, methionine, and tryptophan. Protein is found in meat, fish, eggs, dairy products, beans, maize, peas, nuts and whole-grain cereals.

Fats are required to build and repair cells and to act as chemical messengers to activate body functions. They occur either as saturated or unsaturated fats. Saturated fats in food can be used by the liver to produce CHOLESTEROL, which is implicated in ARTERIOSCLEROSIS, HEART DISEASE and STROKE. Unsaturated fats are regarded as more healthy, but overall the diet should contain less than 30 per cent fat.

Fibre is the part of vegetables, unrefined cereal grains and seeds that the body cannot digest, e.g. bran. Insoluble fibre adds bulk to faeces, preventing CONSTIPATION. Soluble fibre acts to modify the absorption of fats and reduces blood cholesterol. It is recommended that everyone should eat 1 oz (25 g) of fibre each day. Health authorities recommend eating at least 5 portions of fruit and vegetables a day, which provide essential vitamins, minerals, fibre and carbohydrates.

During PREGNANCY a healthy diet is essential. Protein requirement increases by 30 per cent, and extra calories are needed. Higher levels of VITAMINS and minerals are needed to support development of the foetus. Iron, calcium, vitamin B_{12} (cyanocobalamin), folic acid and zinc are all required for formation of tissues and development of the baby. Vegan mothers may need to take vitamin B_{12} supplements as this is present in animal-derived foodstuffs.

O

obesity the accumulation of excess fat in the body, mainly in the subcutaneous tissues, caused by eating more food than is necessary to produce the required energy for each day's activity. The effects of obesity are serious, being associated with increased mortality and illness, including cardiovascular disease, DIABETES, GALL BLADDER complaints, HERNIA, and many others. Treatment involves eating a low energy, balanced diet with more drastic measures (e.g. stapling of the stomach) rarely being necessary.

obsessive-compulsive disorder a condition in which a person's behaviour changes to the point where it disrupts the normal routine of daily life. The most common problems are excessive handwashing and checking something over and over again. The person knows the actions are irrational but still feels compelled to go through the ritual. This disrupts normal relationships, causing guilt, shame and DEPRESSION. The disorder often develops in response to a significant stress, such as PREGNANCY, childbirth, exhaustion, work problems, bereavement or a difficult marriage. Treatment includes discovering the cause of the obsession and gradual moves to change the sufferer's behaviour. The aim is to teach the person to control his or her behaviour and realize that it is not necessary.

obstetrician a doctor who specializes in the care of women during PREGNANCY, DELIVERY and the POSTNATAL period (6 weeks after birth).

oedema an accumulation of fluid in the body, possibly beneath the skin or in cavities or organs. Following an injury the swelling may be localized but is more general in cases of kidney or heart failure. Fluid can collect in the chest cavity, abdomen or lung. The causes are numerous, including liver cirrhosis, starvation, INFLAMMATION of the kidney, allergy or drugs. To alleviate the symptom the root cause has to be removed.

oestrogen a (natural) group of steroid HORMONES that are produced mainly by the ovaries (*see* OVARY) but also in small amounts by the ADRENAL GLANDS and PLACENTA during PREGNANCY. At PUBERTY, the PITUITARY GLAND produces FSH (follicle-stimulating HORMONE) that stimulates the development of ovarian FOLLICLES and oestrogen production. This hormone accounts for the growth of the BREASTS, UTERUS, VAGINA and FALLOPIAN TUBES during puberty and also pubic and underarm hair. Oestrogen also prompts an increase in the proportion of fat in the body and a different pattern of distribution that leads to the characteristic female figure. From puberty through to the MENOPAUSE, there are variable levels of oestrogen in the body according to the time in the MENSTRUAL CYCLE. Small quantities of oestrogen are produced in fatty tissue. ANDROGENS (from the adrenal glands) are converted into oestrogen, and this process continues after the menopause. There are 3 main naturally occurring oestrogens—oestradiol, oestriol and oestrone—and 17 minor forms. Synthetic and naturally occurring oestrogens are used in HORMONE REPLACEMENT THERAPY, the combined ORAL CONTRACEPTIVE PILL and in some other hormone therapies. (*See also* PROGESTERONE.)

oligomenorrhoea infrequent menstrual periods with breaks of 38 or more days in between. It is particularly common at MENARCHE and in the time leading up to the MENOPAUSE. Other causes are emotional problems, severe dieting and OBESITY. Oligomenorrhoea may be a symptom of disease affecting the THYROID or ADRENAL GLAND, and the condition may cause problems if a woman wishes to conceive. (*See also* MENSTRUAL CYCLE.)

oophorectomy the surgical removal of one or both ovaries. It may be carried out to treat OVARIAN CYSTS or OVARIAN CANCER or damage caused by infection such as in PELVIC INFLAMMATORY DISEASE. The removal of both ovaries, UTERUS and FALLOPIAN TUBES often leads to the onset of the MENOPAUSE. (*See also* HYSTERECTOMY.)

oral contraceptive pill one of a number of types of hormonal oral contraceptive pill. The preparations are all forms of the combined OESTROGEN and PROGESTERONE pill or the progesterone-only pill (*see* MINI-PILL). The combined pill was first developed in the 1960s and is the most popular form of CONTRACEPTION overall, largely because of its great effectiveness in preventing pregnancy. It stops OVULATION from taking place, alters the action of the FALLOPIAN TUBES so movement of SPERM and EGG is limited and prevents the ENDOMETRIUM from thickening. This makes it around 97 per cent effective in preventing pregnancy, but it can produce SIDE-EFFECTS, including WEIGHT GAIN, BREAST tenderness, NAUSEA, BREAKTHROUGH BLEEDING, FLUID RETENTION, HEADACHES, dizziness and vaginal discharge. The pill is simple to use, reduces PREMENSTRUAL TENSION, MENSTRUAL FLOW and CRAMPS and regulates the MENSTRUAL CYCLE. With many variations available, a woman can switch brands to minimize any side-effects.

The pill may benefit a woman's health by reducing the risk of ANAEMIA, painful periods, OVARIAN CYSTS, PELVIC INFLAMMATORY DISEASE, FIBROIDS, BENIGN breast disorders (e.g. FIBROADENOMA, SCLEROSING ADENOSIS), and OVARIAN and ENDOMETRIAL CANCER. There may also be a reduction in the risk of RHEUMATOID ARTHRITIS and thyroid diseases. The combined pill is not suitable for every woman and should not be taken by those with certain existing disorders. These are heart and liver disease, previous STROKE, MIGRAINE, DIABETES, GALLSTONES, CYSTIC FIBROSIS, SICKLE-CELL ANAEMIA, HYPERTENSION, or former BREAST or OVARIAN CANCER. The combined pill can exacerbate epilepsy, asthma and kidney disease. Women who are overweight or smoke are regarded at higher risk and may not be prescribed this preparation. All women on the combined pill should be monitored for the first 3–6 months and then have a yearly check-up. The main risk is an increased likelihood of DEEP-VEIN THROMBOSIS, pulmonary embolism, heart disease, STROKE and high BLOOD PRESSURE. There may be an increased risk of breast cancer, but this is not yet fully evaluated. Occasionally women develop CH-LOASMA (pigmentation of the face and neck), DEPRESSION, ANXIETY and MOOD CHANGES, but these generally decline after a few months of use. Some 80–100 million women worldwide use the combined contraceptive pill.

orgasm the climax of SEXUAL AROUSAL in which there is release of congestion and muscle tension leading to a feeling of intense pleasure. The lower VAGINA and surrounding tissue contract along with the UTERUS and PELVIC FLOOR MUSCLES to produce an orgasm. The process and experience of orgasm differs from woman to woman. Some can experience multiple orgasms separated only by a few minutes. Women tend to take longer than men to reach orgasm, but this can vary widely. 'Female ejaculation', which some women experience, can occur if the SKENE'S GLANDS near the urethra secrete fluid upon orgasm. (*See also* SEXUAL AROUSAL; PELVIC CONGESTION.)

osteoarthritis the most common form of ARTHRITIS in which the cartilage between joints degenerates, causing pain and INFLAMMATION. The condition usually develops after the age of 45, and in women several joints are generally affected while in men it is normally one. The hip, knee and finger joints are most frequently affected, impairing their function. The condition can develop because of overuse or strain of joints or because of injury. Normal treatment is with non-steroidal anti-inflammatory drugs, rest, weight loss to lessen strain, ice packs or heat pads to reduce pain and swelling, and EXERCISE such as swimming to increase mobility. In severe cases, hip or knee replacement surgery may be needed, which gives good results. (*See also* RHEUMATOID ARTHRITIS.)

osteoporosis a condition in which the amount of BONE mass decreases to the point where the bones are fragile and easily fractured, affecting twice as many women as men. Normally bone is reabsorbed into the body and replaced by new bone tissue, but after the age of 35 the density starts to fall and loss is greater than replacement, and this process accelerates after the MENOPAUSE. Bone density peaks between 25 and 35 in women, and this requires an adequate supply of calcium and VITAMIN D. Women are at particular risk from osteoporosis as they have a lower density of bone, because of smaller body size, than men. The risk increases in those who have a premature menopause (before 45), early HYSTERECTOMY, previous ANOREXIA NERVOSA or BULIMIA NERVOSA, long-term steroid treatment, AMENORRHOEA because of hormonal irregularities (e.g. POLYCYSTIC OVARIAN SYNDROME) or excessive EXERCISE. Also women who smoke or drink excessively are at greater risk. Exercise appears to slow down bone loss and have a protective effect, as does a diet rich in calcium. The disorder is usually diagnosed when a woman has low backache, loss of height, curvature of the spine or a fractured bone caused by a minor injury or fall, and is confirmed by an X-RAY or bone scan. Weight-bearing exercise, a diet rich in calcium, vitamin D and other minerals, and not smoking can help prevent bone loss. HORMONE REPLACEMENT THERAPY is the most effective preventive treatment but is not suitable for all women. Some drugs can help strengthen specific areas such as the spine and increase bone mass, but they may pose some degree of risk. Physiotherapy and ACUPUNCTURE can help to relieve pain.

otoplasty a type of COSMETIC SURGERY carried out to change the shape of the ear flap, usually to correct protruding ears.

ovarian cancer the growth of MALIGNANT cells in one OVARY or both. It is the fifth most common CANCER in women and one that has a fatality rate of greater than 80 per cent. It mainly affects women after the age of 40, with 90 per cent of cases developing after 45. European and American women appear to have a greater incidence, which may indicate an environmental or dietary factor. Women who have had the maximum number of periods, i.e. who have never been pregnant, are more liable to develop the disease. PREGNANCY, the ORAL CONTRACEPTIVE PILL and STERILIZATION all seem to have protective effects. The disease is difficult to detect early as few symptoms appear. PELVIC PAIN, abdominal swelling, weight loss, NAUSEA and changes in bowel or urinary habits may occur but generally only later in the course of the disease. BLOOD TESTS and ULTRASOUND can detect a tumour, and tests are carried out to determine the presence of cancer. If caught early when only the ovaries are affected, surgical removal can be an effective treatment. However, only 15 per cent of ovarian cancer is found at this point. Once the cancer has invaded the abdomen, more extensive surgery and CHEMO-THERAPY are needed, and 20 per cent of women survive for 10 years or more.

Some new drugs and monoclonal antibodies that directly target the cancer cells may offer more effective treatment with a higher success rate. Screening of women with a family history of the disease is likely to prove helpful as there appears to be an hereditary factor involved. After bilateral OOPHORECTOMY, HORMONE REPLACE-MENT THERAPY may be needed to relieve menopausal symptoms. Women with ovarian cancer have a far higher risk (4 times greater) of developing BREAST CANCER and vice versa.

ovarian cyst a CYST that develops in the OVARY and can be BENIGN or MALIGNANT. Cysts can arise at any age in one or both ovaries, either singly or in multiples. Many ovarian cysts are termed 'functional', i.e. they develop because of normal functioning of the ovary during the MENSTRUAL CYCLE. If an ovarian FOLLICLE fails to release an EGG it can become a cyst, as can the CORPUS LUTEUM if it is not reabsorbed as normal. These cysts usually disappear after one or two menstrual cycles. Ovarian cysts do not normally cause symptoms until they increase in size to sufficient extent to be felt by PELVIC EXAMINATION. Common symptoms are abdominal swelling, change in pattern of MENSTRUAL CYCLE, increased frequency of urination, breathlessness, INFERTILITY, AMENORRHOEA and PAINFUL IN-TERCOURSE. In rare cases the cyst may twist, stopping its blood supply and resulting in severe abdominal pain that requires emergency surgery. The presence of a cyst can be confirmed by ULTRASOUND, and surgical investigation is required to determine the presence of malignancy. This usually involves LAPAROSCOPY and BIOPSY of a tumour sample. A benign cyst can be removed surgically and the ovary repaired, but if it is cancerous, the whole ovary and FALLOPIAN TUBE are normally removed. The second ovary is also examined and removed if necessary.

ovarian follicle *see* FOLLICLE, OVARIAN.

ovary one of a pair of female GONADS (sex organs) that are primarily responsible for producing the female GAMETES (EGGS or ova) and

the hormones OESTROGEN and PROGESTERONE. Each ovary is about
the size of an almond and located one on either side of the UTERUS.
In each MENSTRUAL CYCLE, one (or two) egg develops inside a GRAA-
FIAN FOLLICLE and is released at OVULATION. If an egg is fertilized by
a SPERM and the EMBRYO implants in the uterus, PREGNANCY begins.
After the MENOPAUSE, any remaining eggs degenerate, and the ovary
shrinks in size. The most common conditions affecting the ovaries
are OVARIAN CYSTS and OVARIAN CANCER, but they can also become
infected in PELVIC INFLAMMATORY DISEASE and some SEXUALLY TRANS-
MITTED DISEASES. As surgical removal of the ovaries (OOPHORECTOMY)
hastens the menopause, it is used only as a treatment of last resort
when other methods have failed. (*See also* FOLLICLE.)

oviducts an alternative name for FALLOPIAN TUBES, used to describe
these structures in vertebrate animals.

ovulation the release of a mature EGG from a GRAAFIAN FOLLICLE in
the OVARY. Ovulation is triggered by secretion of LH (luteinizing hormone) from the PITUITARY GLAND. (*See also* MENSTRUAL CYCLE, FOL-
LICLE.)

ovum *see* EGG.

oxytocin a HORMONE that is stored and released by the PITUITARY
GLAND under control of the HYPOTHALAMUS. It acts to stimulate uterine CONTRACTIONS during LABOUR and causes contraction of the cells
lining the milk ducts in the BREAST, so expelling milk. A synthetic
form is used to induce labour and to strengthen weak contractions.
Its use must be carefully controlled as it may cause severe contractions that can be dangerous to the baby and painful to the mother.
(*See also* ABORTION; INDUCTION OF LABOUR; LET-DOWN REFLEX.)

P

Paget's disease of the nipple a rare form of BREAST CANCER in
which the NIPPLE and AREOLA look encrusted. The cause is CANCER
affecting the milk ducts, and it occurs most often in middle-aged
women.

Paget's disease of bone (osteitis deformans) a CHRONIC disease, particularly affecting the long bones, skull and spine, that results in them becoming thickened, disorganized and also soft, causing bending. The main symptom is pain. The cause is unknown, and although there is no cure, good results are being obtained with the HORMONE calcitonin.

painful intercourse *see* DYSPAREUNIA.

painful urination *see* DYSURIA.

palpitation a situation in which the heart beats noticeably or irregularly and the person becomes aware of it doing so. The heartbeat is not normally noticed, but with fear, emotion or EXERCISE it may be felt, causing an unpleasant sensation. Palpitations may also be due to neuroses, arrhythmia or HEART DISEASE, and a common cause is too much tea, coffee, ALCOHOL or smoking. Where an excess is the cause (tea, coffee, etc), this can be eliminated. For disease-associated palpitations, drugs can be used for control.

pancreas a GLAND with both ENDOCRINE and exocrine functions. It is located between the duodenum and spleen, behind the stomach, and is about 15 cm long. There are 2 types of cells producing secretions, one being the ACINI, which secrete pancreatic juice that goes to the intestine via a system of ducts. This contains an alkaline mixture of salt and enzymes—trypsin and chymotrypsin to digest proteins, amylase to break down starch, and lipase to aid digestion of fats. The second cell types are in the Islets of Langerhans, and these produce 2 HORMONES, insulin and glucagon, secreted directly into the BLOOD for control of sugar levels (*see* DIABETES).

panic attack *see* ANXIETY.

Pap smear an alternative name for CERVICAL SMEAR TEST.

parathyroid glands four ENDOCRINE GLANDS located behind the THYROID GLAND in the neck. They produce parathyroid HORMONE, which regulates the use of calcium and phosphorus in the body.

parturition childbirth (*see* DELIVERY; LABOUR).

pelvic and abdominal pain pain in the pelvic region, often from the reproductive organs. Pelvic pain is a symptom that results from various conditions, including PELVIC INFLAMMATORY DISEASE, OVARIAN CYSTS, PELVIC CONGESTION, ENDOMETRIOSIS, FIBROIDS and ECTOPIC

PREGNANCY, and MISCARRIAGE. INFLAMMATION of the appendix (AP-
PENDICITIS), ovaries, ENDOMETRIUM, bowel or intestine may cause
pain in the pelvis, as can CYSTITIS, urinary tract infections,
OSTEOARTHRITIS, or OSTEOPOROSIS affecting the lower back. This type
of pain may result from a slipped disc in the back, poor posture,
SCOLIOSIS or a tumour in the BONE, ovaries or CERVIX. Other conditions that cause severe abdominal pain include perforation, obstruction or rupture of organs, as in a strangulated hernia or burst appendix.

pelvic cancer a general term for CANCER of the reproductive organs
in the PELVIS, in particular the UTERUS, (CERVIX and ENDOMETRIUM),
OVARIES, FALLOPIAN TUBES, VAGINA and VULVA.

pelvic congestion a painful condition in which the BLOOD vessels in
the PELVIS become enlarged and congested. Pain may be intermittent or continual and can be triggered by SEXUAL INTERCOURSE, prolonged standing or by STRESS. Treatment is by taking synthetic PRO-
GESTERONE and measures to control stress. In very severe cases and
where no other cure is possible, HYSTERECTOMY and OOPHORECTOMY
may be carried out. Pelvic congestion is not widely recognized by
doctors.

pelvic examination a routine check of internal pelvic organs. Normally, the woman lies on her back with her knees raised and legs
apart. The external GENITALS may be checked if necessary but internal structures are examined by placing two gloved fingers in the
VAGINA with the other hand placed on top of the abdomen (bi-
manual examination). This allows a doctor to assess size, shape,
position and tenderness of the UTERUS, ovaries and FALLOPIAN TUBES.
A SPECULUM may be inserted into the vagina so that the vaginal
walls and CERVIX can be viewed to check for any swelling, irritation
or redness. A CERVICAL SMEAR TEST may be taken and other samples
if appropriate. A pelvic examination is carried out before prescribing any form of CONTRACEPTION and to investigate vaginal discharge,
INFECTION or unusual bleeding, and menstrual irregularities. It is
normally carried out at some stage in PREGNANCY. This examination may be done if a woman thinks she has a SEXUALLY TRANSMIT-
TED DISEASE or if her mother took DES (diethylstilboestrol). A pel-

vic examination may be slightly uncomfortable, but it is needed for the DIAGNOSIS of any pelvic problems and as a part of preventive health care. (*See also* GYNAECOLOGICAL EXAMINATION.)

pelvic floor muscles two groups of muscles situated around the URETHRA, VAGINA and anus and supporting the BLADDER, bowel and UTERUS. These muscles can be strengthened by completing KEGEL EXERCISES each day, helping to prevent PROLAPSE and urinary INCONTINENCE.

pelvic inflammatory disease (PID) INFLAMMATION of the FALLOPIAN TUBES, ovaries and UTERUS. The disease can be ACUTE or CHRONIC. Acute PID causes severe ABDOMINAL PAIN, high FEVER, chills, foul-smelling vaginal discharge and abdominal tenderness. Frequently ADHESIONS form between pelvic organs and the intestines or rectum, which can be extremely painful. A PELVIC EXAMINATION and laboratory analysis of the discharge aid DIAGNOSIS. A complication in both acute and chronic PID is the formation of an ABSCESS that may need surgical drainage. If it bursts, it can cause infection of the entire pelvic and abdominal cavity (peritonitis). Blood poisoning (septicaemia) or filling of a Fallopian tube with fluid (hydrosalpinx) that may cause it to burst, are other possible complications of acute PID. However, these are rare as severe pain causes most women to seek prompt medical attention.

PID is the result of bacterial INFECTION, but CHLAMYDIA and GONORRHOEA are responsible for many cases. *Escherichia coli* and the tuberculosis bacterium can also cause PID. Treatment is by means of antibiotics and bed rest. The condition usually improves within 2 weeks but, if not, another antibiotic is given. If 3 courses of antibiotics do not clear the infection, then the disease is deemed to have become chronic. Chronic PID results in a low level of infection that can continue for weeks or months.

Symptoms are persistent abdominal pain or cramps, FATIGUE, weakness and very heavy menstrual periods. Some mild cases have few or no symptoms but can cause partial or total INFERTILITY. Even in a mild form, adhesions may form and distort the Fallopian tubes, changing their shape or sealing their open end, so affecting FERTILITY. Partial blockage of a tube leads to a higher risk of ECTOPIC

PREGNANCY, and the scar tissue can cause severe pain during SEXUAL INTERCOURSE and menstrual periods. Some cases of chronic PID do not respond well to bed rest and oral antibiotics, and severe infections may only be resolved by surgery to remove adhesions, or even the reproductive organs. INTRAUTERINE DEVICE use increases the risk of contracting PID, as does a D AND C, ABORTION or DELIVERY of a baby. The use of CONDOMS and DIAPHRAGMS helps prevent the spread of all sexually transmitted infections. PID can recur, and any abnormal vaginal discharge should always be investigated.

pelvimetry the process of measuring a woman's PELVIS to determine the size of the BIRTH CANAL and to judge if vaginal DELIVERY of a baby is possible.

pelvis the skeletal structure formed by the hip bones, sacrum and coccyx and connects with the spine and legs. The female pelvis is shallower and the ilia are wider apart, and there are certain angular differences compared to the male, all of which relate to childbearing. The pelvis is a point of contact for the muscles of the legs, and it partially envelops the BLADDER and RECTUM. In females it contains the UTERUS and ovaries.

perineum muscles, fibrous tissue and skin between the anus and the VAGINA. It is this area that stretches, thins and tears to allow passage of a baby to the outside and that is cut if an EPISIOTOMY is needed to enlarge the vaginal opening.

pessary an instrument that fits into the VAGINA to treat a PROLAPSE. Also, a soft solid that is shaped for insertion into the vagina and contains drugs for some gynaecological disorder (also used for inducing labour).

phenylketonuria a genetic disorder that results in the deficiency of an enzyme that converts phenylalanine, an essential amino acid, to tyrosine. Children can be severely mentally retarded by an excess of phenylalanine in the BLOOD damaging the NERVOUS SYSTEM. The responsible GENE is recessive so the condition occurs only if both parents are carriers. However, there is a test for newborn infants (the Guthrie test) that ensures the condition can be detected and the diet can be modified to avoid phenylalanine and thus any brain damage.

phlebitis INFLAMMATION of VEINS, most commonly those in the legs and pelvic area. It affects superficial veins rather than larger, deeper ones (*compare* DEEP-VEIN THROMBOSIS) and often accompanies VARICOSE VEINS. Generally, part of the vein becomes painful and tender and appears as a red streak on the skin. A THROMBUS (BLOOD CLOT) causes the coloration by fixing to the vein wall, but there is no risk of an embolus breaking away, as in deep-vein thrombosis. Treatment is by bed rest, elevation of the leg and wearing elastic support stockings to prevent FLUID RETENTION. If there is INFECTION, antibiotics are given and also blood-thinning agents.

Phyllodes tumour a rare BREAST tumour that is usually BENIGN and generally develops between the ages of 35 and 55. It is related to FIBROADENOMA and may accompany this condition. Phyllodes tumours are soft and can grow large enough to fill the whole breast. They can recur so surgical removal is usually carried out, and this can necessitate a simple MASTECTOMY because of the size of the tumour. BREAST PLASTIC SURGERY may then be needed.

pica an abnormal desire to eat non-food substances such as soap, chalk, glue, clay, etc. The disorder may arise during early childhood or in mental illness. Although it also occurs during PREGNANCY, the desire is more often for unusual foods and an excess of ordinary foods. In some cases pica may result from a mineral deficiency in the body.

PID *see* PELVIC INFLAMMATORY DISEASE.

pineal gland a structure found in the brain that produces the HORMONE melatonin, responsible for skin pigmentation. It may act to initiate development of the GONADS, but this is not certain.

pituitary gland a small but very important ENDOCRINE GLAND at the base of the HYPOTHALAMUS. The pituitary secretes HORMONES that control many functions and is itself controlled by hormonal secretions from the hypothalamus. One lobe of the gland stores and releases peptide hormones produced in the hypothalamus, namely OXYTOCIN and vasopressin, and the other secretes the growth hormone gonadotrophin, PROLACTIN, adrenocorticotrophic hormone (ACTH) and thyroid-stimulating hormones.

placenta the organ attaching the EMBRYO to the UTERUS. It is a temporary feature comprising maternal and embryonic tissues, and it allows oxygen and nutrients to pass from the mother's BLOOD to the embryo's blood. There is, however, no direct contact of blood supplies. The embryo also receives salt, glucose, amino acids, some peptides and ANTIBODIES, fats and VITAMINS. Waste molecules from the embryo are removed by diffusion into the maternal circulation. The placenta also stores glycogen, for conversion to glucose if required, and secretes HORMONES to regulate the PREGNANCY. It is expelled after birth in the third stage of LABOUR.

placenta praevia a rare condition in which the PLACENTA is situated in the bottom part of the UTERUS next to or over the CERVIX. This results in bleeding with no pain, either late in PREGNANCY (8 months onwards) or during LABOUR and can be diagnosed using ULTRASOUND. The main risk is PREMATURE BIRTH and HAEMORRHAGE in the mother. Depending on the severity of the condition, vaginal DELIVERY may be possible, but 60 per cent of cases require a CAESAREAN SECTION to reduce risks to the mother and baby. The chance of placenta praevia developing increases with age and number of previous pregnancies. (*See also* ABRUPTIO PLACENTAE).

polycystic ovarian syndrome a condition in which one OVARY or both has multiple small CYSTS. Recent screening has found that at least 20 per cent of all women have polycystic ovaries but mostly without the characteristic symptoms, which include OBESITY, irregular MENSTRUAL CYCLES or AMENORRHOEA and HIRSUTISM. The syndrome is thought to be caused by an imbalance of FSH (follicle-stimulating hormone) and LH (luteinizing hormone), produced by the PITUITARY GLAND, that leads to an increase in the male hormones, ANDROGENS. Treatment may be by administering anti-androgen drugs, the combined ORAL CONTRACEPTIVE PILL or drugs to suppress the ovaries. These have limited success but losing weight, if obese, and taking EXERCISE can also help resolve the condition.

polymenorrhoea a regular MENSTRUAL CYCLE of fewer than 22 days. There may be excessive bleeding, possibly leading to ANAEMIA. It is often caused by hormonal imbalance or possibly FIBROIDS.

polyps soft growths of tissue that can develop in the ENDOMETRIUM or CERVIX. They may cause no symptoms or there may be intermittent bleeding, particularly after SEXUAL INTERCOURSE. They are detected by PELVIC EXAMINATION or HYSTEROSCOPY and are removed by CAUTERIZATION or a D AND C. Polyps can recur and rarely become MALIGNANT. (*See also* CERVICAL POLYP.)

postmature a baby born after the 42nd week of GESTATION. The baby may be unharmed or may be underweight because of placental failure and insufficient supply of nutrients and oxygen, which can occur in a prolonged PREGNANCY.

postmenopausal bleeding bleeding or staining in a woman past the MENOPAUSE. The bleeding may be a sign of serious disorder such as CANCER or result from surgery or HORMONE REPLACEMENT THERAPY. The cause must always be investigated and established.

postnatal care the care of the mother after childbirth. After a HOSPITAL BIRTH, a woman is discharged within 24 hours or after 2–3 days as long as there are no problems. Before this she is examined to check that the UTERUS is decreasing in size, stitches are healing and that the LOCHIA shows no sign of INFECTION. Advice about CONTRACEPTION and routine baby care are given and a date for a postnatal check-up. This is usually 6 weeks after the birth and may include a PELVIC EXAMINATION and discussion about the mother's state of health. Pain during the postnatal period may indicate infection and should be investigated. Community midwives visit the mother and baby for several days in her own home, and the family doctor is also in close attendance so that any early problems are usually detected. Most family doctors also give the mother a postnatal check-up. (*See also* POSTNATAL DEPRESSION; POSTPARTUM HAEMORRHAGE; PUERPERAL FEVER).

postnatal depression DEPRESSION that occurs after childbirth. It may be caused by the rapid change in HORMONE levels after the birth or by the birth experience itself, especially if this did not meet expectations. Symptoms include irritability, extreme FATIGUE, INSOMNIA, ANXIETY, hopelessness, guilt, lack of concentration and self-esteem, panic and obsessional thoughts. Prompt sympathetic treatment is vital, and ANTIDEPRESSANT drugs may be needed with rest, gentle EXERCISE, a good diet, support and help with the baby and talking about the depression. Recovery may take some time. This form of depression can spoil the mother's enjoyment of her new baby and make BONDING more difficult.

postpartum the initial period after childbirth, lasting 2–3 days. It is similar to POSTNATAL but usually refers to a longer period of time.

postpartum haemorrhage heavy bleeding after childbirth, which usually occurs because there is placental tissue remaining in the UTERUS. This requires a D AND C to remove the tissue and possibly a BLOOD transfusion and iron supplements.

precancerous a term to describe any condition that is not MALIGNANT but will become so if left untreated.

precocious puberty sexual development and menstrual periods in girls before the age of 8 or 9. It results from premature signals from the HYPOTHALAMUS, pituitary and ADRENAL GLANDS, which trigger PUBERTY.

pre-eclampsia the development of high BLOOD PRESSURE in PREGNANCY, sometimes with OEDEMA, that, unless treated, may result in ECLAMPSIA.

pregnancy the period of time from CONCEPTION to DELIVERY, whichlasts approximately 280 days from the first day of the last menstrual period (LMP). Pregnancy continues for 9 months or 39–40 weeks and is divided into three TRIMESTERS. Signs of pregnancy are AMENORRHOEA or cessation of periods, MORNING SICKNESS, increased BREAST size and later enlargement of the abdomen. In the first trimester, the EMBRYO implants, grows and develops. HORMONE levels rise, and the BLOOD supply to the PELVIS increases, resulting in CHANDWICK'S SIGN. The baby's heartbeat can be detected at 11 weeks' GESTATION. In the second trimester the size and shape of the UTERUS has changed, and there may be signs on the mother's skin such as pigment changes (CHLOASMA) or STRETCH MARKS. The woman commonly has a faster heart rate, increased blood volume and may have VARICOSE VEINS, HAEMORRHOIDS, OEDEMA and breathlessness. The large size of the uterus by the third trimester can lead to discomfort and pressure on the other body organs. Indigestion, CONSTIPATION, FATIGUE, heartburn and urinary frequency are common. Good ANTENATAL CARE can guide the woman through these problems and prepare her and her partner for LABOUR. (*See also* HIGH-RISK PREGNANCY; PREGNANCY PROBLEMS).

pregnancy problems these can include abdominal and PELVIC PAIN, BACKACHE, leg CRAMPS, CONSTIPATION, FAINTING, INSOMNIA, FLUID RETENTION, cravings (PICA), HAEMORRHOIDS, heartburn, STRESS INCONTINENCE, MORNING SICKNESS, CHLOASMA, rib pain, tiredness, STRETCH MARKS, night sweats and VARICOSE VEINS.

pregnancy test a BLOOD or URINE TEST to detect HUMAN CHORIONIC GONADOTROPIN, which, if positive, indicates CONCEPTION has occurred. Some can be carried out at home (urine tests) but usually a sample is sent to a laboratory.

premature birth one occurring before full term. The definition refers to babies weighing less than 2 kg. In many cases the cause is unknown, but may be due to PRE-ECLAMPSIA, kidney or HEART DISEASE or MULTIPLE PREGNANCY. Premature babies often require incubator care.

premenstrual tension the occurrence for up to 10 days before the MENSTRUAL CYCLE of such symptoms as HEADACHE, nervousness and irritability, emotional disturbance, DEPRESSION, FATIGUE, with other physical manifestations such as swelling of legs and BREASTS, and CONSTIPATION. The condition usually disappears soon after menstruation begins. The cause is not known although the hormone PROGESTERONE is probably involved in some way.

prenatal care *see* ANTENATAL CARE.

prepared childbirth preparing for LABOUR and DELIVERY by learning about the birth process and the various exercises and breathing techniques that can be useful. The aim is to prepare the parents thoroughly, particularly the mother, about what could happen during labour and delivery. It may take the form of antenatal classes run by midwives at theGP's surgery and hospital or by other organizations, especially the Natural Childbirth Trust.

primigravida a woman who is pregnant for the first time.

primipara a woman who has given birth to one child.

progesterone a steroid HORMONE that is vital in PREGNANCY. It is produced by the CORPUS LUTEUM of the OVARY when the lining of the UTERUS is prepared for the implanting of a fertilized EGG cell. Progesterone is secreted under the control of other hormones (PROLACTIN and LH from the PITUITARY GLAND) until the PLACENTA adopts this role later in the pregnancy. The function of progesterone is to maintain the uterus and ensure no further eggs are produced. Small amounts of this hormone are also produced by the testes. (*See also* MENSTRUAL CYCLE; MINI-PILL.)

prognosis a forecast of the likely outcome of a disease based on the patient's state of health and the history of the condition in other patients.

prolactin a HORMONE produced by the PITUITARY GLAND that stimulates the production of BREAST milk after childbirth and encourages secretion of PROGESTERONE by the CORPUS LUTEUM. Excess prolactin gives rise to GALACTORRHOEA. (*See also* BREAST-FEEDING; LETDOWN REFLEX.)

prolapse a moving down of an organ or tissue from its normal position because of weakening of the supporting tissue. This may happen to the lower end of the bowel (in children) or the UTERUS and VAGINA in women who have sustained some sort of injury during childbirth. In the latter case prolapse may result in the uterus itself protruding to the outside of the body. Surgery can be carried out to shorten the supporting ligaments and narrow the vaginal opening. (*See also* CYSTOCELE; RECTOCELE; URETHROCELE.)

prolapsed cord a situation in childbirth in which the UMBILICAL CORD comes through the CERVIX before the baby. If the cord is compressed, the baby's oxygen supply can be affected with possibly fatal results. If the cervix is fully dilated, immediate vaginal DELIVERY of the baby is needed to save its life. Otherwise an emergency CAESAREAN SECTION is required.

prolonged labour LABOUR that lasts for longer than the normal time. This may be due to ABNORMAL PRESENTATION, weak uterine CONTRACTIONS or a pelvis that is is too small for the baby to pass through. Prolonged labour tends to occur in women aged over 35, with a large baby and in first time births.

prophylactic some treatment or action that is taken to avoid disease or a condition, e.g. taking a medication to prevent angina.

prostaglandin (PG) a group of compounds derived from essential fatty acids that act in a similar way to HORMONES. They are found in most body tissues, where they are released as local regulators (in the UTERUS, brain, lungs, etc). A number have been identified, two of which act antagonistically on blood vessels: PGE causing dilation, PGF constriction. Certain prostaglandins cause uterine CONTRACTION in LABOUR (and are used to induce abortion), and others are involved in the body's defence mechanisms.

pruritis vulvae ITCHING of the skin around the GENITALS and anus, particularly the VULVA. It can be due to a VAGINAL INFECTION, e.g. THRUSH, MENOPAUSE, allergy, DIABETES or PUBIC LICE.

psychotherapy a type of counselling or therapy in which the patient discusses his or her problems with a psychotherapist. It is used to help mental and emotional disorders.

puberty the period during which sexual maturity is gained. In girls it usually starts between the ages of 10 and 18 and lasts for about 5 years. There is a period of WEIGHT GAIN and growth in height, and MENARCHE occurs because of the hormones OESTROGEN and PROGESTERONE. The pattern of fat deposition changes, producing the characteristic female body shape, the UTERUS enlarges, and the GENITALS develop and mature. The secondary sexual characteristics develop with growth of underarm and PUBIC HAIR, enlargement of BREASTS and sweat glands.

On rare occasions puberty starts before age 9 (PRECOCIOUS PUBERTY) or may fail completely, usually because of disorders of the PITUITARY GLAND or ovaries.

pubic hair hair that grows over the genital area during PUBERTY.

pubic or **crab lice** are insect parasites that can be transmitted by infected clothing or bedding or by sexual contact. They feed on blood and lay numerous eggs throughout their 30-day lifespan. They cause severe itching in the genital region and are treated with insecticidal creams such as malathion. Clothing and bedding also need to be treated and washed, heated or incinerated.

pubococcygeous the muscle in the pelvic floor that supports the UTERUS, BLADDER and RECTUM. This muscle is used to stop the flow of URINE and can be strengthened by KEGEL EXERCISES. The PELVIC FLOOR MUSCLES can be weakened after childbirth, leading to STRESS INCONTINENCE and PROLAPSE.

puerperal fever an INFECTION, now rare in developed countries, that

occurs within 2–3 days of childbirth when a mother is susceptible
to disease. Since the body's resources are low and the genital tract
after childbirth provides ready access for bacteria, it is essential
that clean conditions are maintained to avoid infection. A mild infection of the genital tract may cause FEVER, high temperature and
pulse. INFLAMMATION and possibly peritonitis may result from infection of local LYMPH and BLOOD vessels while access to the general
circulation can cause septicaemia. Serious cases are, however, rare.
Preventive measures are vital, but infections respond to antibiotic
treatment.

puerperium the name for the period after childbirth (*compare* POST-
PARTUM, POSTNATAL).

pyelonephritis INFLAMMATION of the part of the kidney from which
URINE drains into the URETER. The cause is usually a bacterial IN-
FECTION (commonly *Escherichia coli*) and sometimes occurs as a
complication of PREGNANCY. The symptoms include pain in the loins,
high temperature and loss of weight, and treatment is by antibiotics.

Q

quickening the first movements of a baby in the WOMB that are perceived by the mother, usually around the 4th month of PREGNANCY.

R

radioreceptor assay a very sensitive pregnancy test that is 99 per
cent accurate.

radiotherapy the therapeutic use of penetrating radiation, including
X-RAYS, beta rays and gamma rays. These may be derived from X-
ray machines or radioactive isotopes and are especially employed
in the treatment of CANCER. The main disadvantage is that there
may be damage to normal, healthy surrounding tissues.

Raynaud's disease a condition in which the arteries in the fingers and toes go into spasm when the hands or feet are cold. The fingers turn white when BLOOD flow through the arteries is reduced, then, when the oxygen supply is used up, the skin goes blue. Finally, the red colour returns as the temperature rises and the blood flow returns to normal. The disease is common in young adults and can be helped by drugs to dilate the blood vessels.

rectocele prolapse of the wall of the RECTUM into the VAGINA, which may occur with CYSTOCELE and a prolapsed uterus. It can be caused by childbirth and is rectified by minor surgery.

rectum the final portion of the large intestine between the colon and anal canal in which faeces are stored prior to elimination.

red blood cell (erythrocyte) a BLOOD cell that is made in the BONE MARROW and occurs as a red disc, concave on both sides, full of HAEMOGLOBIN. These cells are responsible for carrying oxygen to tissues and carbon dioxide away. The latter is removed in the form of the bicarbonate ion ($HCO3^-$), in exchange for a chloride ion (Cl^-). There are approximately five million erythrocytes in one millilitre of blood, and they are active for about 120 days before being absorbed by white blood cells.

remission a period during the course of a disease when symptoms have lessened or disappeared.

respiratory distress syndrome a condition arising in newborn babies, especially those who are PREMATURE, being particularly common in infants born between 32–37 weeks GESTATION. It is also known as hyaline membrane disease and is characterized by rapid shallow laboured breathing. It arises because the lungs are not properly expanded and lack a substance (known as surfactant) necessary to expand the tiny air sacs. In adults the condition is called adult respiratory distress syndrome (ARDS).

retroflexed uterus a UTERUS that doubles back upon itself (see RETROVERTED UTERUS).

retroverted uterus a condition in which the UTERUS is tilted backwards in relation to the VAGINA. It can be present from birth or develop as a result of childbirth. The condition may cause symptoms and hinder CONCEPTION in some women.

rheumatoid arthritis the second most common form of joint disease after OSTEOARTHRITIS, usually affecting the feet, ankles, fingers and wrists. It is diagnosed by means of X-RAYS, which show a typical pattern of changes around the inflamed joints, known as rheumatoid erosions. At first there is swelling of the joint and INFLAMMATION of the synovial membrane (the membraneous sac that surrounds the joint) followed by erosion and loss of cartilage and BONE. In addition, a BLOOD TEST reveals the presence of serum rheumatoid factor ANTIBODY, which is characteristic of this condition. The condition varies greatly in its degree of severity but at its worst can be progressive and seriously disabling. In other people, after an initial active phase, there may be a long period of REMISSION. A number of different drugs are used to treat the disease, including ANALGESICS and anti-inflammatory agents.

rhesus factor (Rh factor) an ANTIGEN present in 85 per cent of the population, who are said to be rhesus positive (Rh+). If it is absent, the blood is rhesus negative (Rh-). If a Rh- woman carries a Rh+ FOETUS her body may produce ANTIBODIES that attack the Rh+ blood cells of the baby. This is called RHESUS INCOMPATIBILITY.

rhesus incompatibility a condition of pregnancy in which a rhesus-negative woman's body produces ANTIBODIES to the RED BLOOD CELLS of her FOETUS, which has rhesus positive BLOOD. This can cause a disease called haemolytic disease of the newborn, in which large amounts of red blood cells are broken down, causing JAUNDICE, blood abnormalities, enlargement of the spleen and liver, and pallor. The baby requires a blood transfusion either after birth or while still in the UTERUS. Not all women become sensitized to Rh+ blood, but all Rh- women are normally given a Rhogham injection to prevent the antibodies from being formed, following an ABORTION, childbirth, AMNIOCENTESIS, CHORIONIC VILLUS SAMPLING or UMBILICAL VEIN SAMPLING.

ripe cervix a softening of the CERVIX that generally occurs near the end of a full-term PREGNANCY.

rubella *see* GERMAN MEASLES.

S

safe sex *see* AIDS.

salpingectomy the surgical removal of one or both FALLOPIAN TUBES.

salpingitis INFLAMMATION and/or INFECTION of the FALLOPIAN TUBES.

Schiller test a test in which the vaginal walls and CERVIX are coated with iodine to isolate abnormal cells. It is used to diagnose VAGINAL or CERVICAL CANCER.

schizophrenia any one of a large group of severe mental disorders typified by gross distortion of reality, disturbance in language and breakdown of thought processes, perceptions and emotions. Delusions and hallucinations are usual, as are apathy, confusion, INCONTINENCE and strange behaviour. No single cause is known, but genetic and biochemical factors are probably important. Drug therapy has improved the outlook markedly over recent years.

sclerosing adenosis a BENIGN LESION or growth found in the BREAST tissue of women of CHILDBEARING AGE. The ACINI tissue becomes distorted, and it is usually treated by surgical removal.

scoliosis progressive lateral curvature of the spine, which is more common in females and often begins in childhood. It may begin in PUBERTY and leads to contraction of the ribs, affecting the lungs and heart and restricting breathing and circulation. It can also be caused by severe chest diseases such as tuberculosis. If not treated by means of surgery or wearing a brace, it can cause invalidism and death.

sex differentiation the process by which the physical characteristics of males and females develop, beginning at FERTILIZATION and continuing until the end of PUBERTY. The normal male sex CHROMOSOMES are XY and female ones are XX. In some cases abnormalities of the sex chromosomes can occur or there may be a defect in HORMONE balance. This can lead to unusual sex chromosome complements, such as XXY, XXX or XYY, which cause the disorders of KLINEFELTER'S SYNDROME or TURNER'S SYNDROME. (*See also* X-CHROMOSOME; Y-CHROMOSOME.)

sexual arousal the physiological process that occurs in women and men after PUBERTY as a result of sexual stimulation of some kind. Research in the 1960s found that it was split into four phases: excitement, plateau, ORGASM, and resolution. These have variable duration and happen as a continuum of increasing (then declining) sexual response. Physical response to sexual arousal is controlled by the NERVOUS SYSTEM and involves involuntary muscles.

sexual intercourse the common name for COITUS, vaginal sex with the man's penis inside the woman's VAGINA.

sexually transmitted disease any INFECTION that is transmitted by sexual contact between partners. The main diseases are AIDS, GONORRHOEA, SYPHILIS, GENITAL HERPES, HEPATITIS, CHLAMYDIA, PUBIC LICE and TRICHOMONAS. Also, THRUSH, CYSTITIS and nonspecific URETHRITIS or VAGINITIS can all be transmitted by sexual contact.

sickle-cell anaemia a type of inherited, haemolytic ANAEMIA that is genetically determined and affects people of African ancestry. It is caused by a recessive GENE and is manifested when this is inherited from both parents.

One amino acid in the HAEMOGLOBIN molecule is substituted, causing the disease, which results in an abnormal type of haemoglobin being precipitated in the RED BLOOD CELLS during deprivation of oxygen. This produces the distortion of the cells, which are removed from the circulation, causing anaemia and JAUNDICE. Many people are carriers because of inheritance of just one defective gene, and since this situation happens to confer increased resistance to malaria, the gene remains at a high level. If this were not the case, it is likely that the defective gene would be less common.

side-effect the additional and unwanted effect(s) of a drug above the intended action. Sometimes side-effects are harmful and may be stronger than anticipated results of the drug, or something quite different.

Sims-Huhner test a postcoital test used to determine SPERM activity in the CERVICAL MUCUS, normally carried out as part of investigations to determine why a couple are having difficulty in conceiving. Around the time of OVULATION the woman is asked to go to the clinic within 2–15 hours of intercourse. She is examined, and a sample of the cervical mucus is removed and examined under a microscope. This can show if the cervical mucus is hostile to her partner's sperm.

Sitz bath a specially designed bath with separate compartments that can be filled with water to a depth of 6 inches and may be used for soaking the hips and genital area. Various medications can be added. It is an effective treatment for CYSTITIS and VAGINITIS, if used several times a day.

Skene's glands a pair of GLANDS located below the female URETHRA of unknown function. They are thought to be the equivalent of the male prostate gland and may produce the female 'ejaculation' in some women. They can develop CYSTS and provide an environment for the bacteria that cause GONORRHOEA.

skin cancer a common type of CANCER of which there are three main types. Basal cell carcinoma and squamous cell carcinoma are usually caused by excessive exposure to the sun and ultraviolet light. They occur most often on the face, neck and the back of the hands, and are readily cured if treated early as they rarely spread. They can be treated by CAUTERIZATION, surgery, radiation or CRYOSURGERY. MALIGNANT melanoma occurs in 5 per cent of skin cancer cases and can spread very quickly. Early detection and treatment ensure success but the cancer can recur. It is wise to reduce exposure to the sun, particularly in childhood, wear protective clothing and a hat, and use sunscreen preparations.

speculum an instrument used to examine the inside of the VAGINA and the CERVIX. It holds the vaginal walls apart so a CERVICAL SMEAR TEST, endometrial BIOPSY, COLOPSCOPY, vaginal HYSTERECTOMY, VACUUM ASPIRATION or D AND C can be performed.

sperm the mature male reproductive cell, or GAMETE. It has a head with a haploid nucleus containing half the CHROMOSOME number, and an acrosome (a structure that aids penetration of the egg). Behind the head there is a midpiece with energy-producing mitochondria and then a long tail that propels it forward. A few millilitres of semen is ejaculated during SEXUAL INTERCOURSE, containing many millions of sperm, only one of which will fertilize an EGG.

spermicide a cream, foam, jelly, etc, that kills SPERM and is used alone or in conjunction with a DIAPHRAGM as a contraceptive.

spina bifida a congenital NEURAL TUBE DEFECT in newborn babies in which part of the spinal cord is exposed by a gap in the backbone. Many babies are also affected with hydrocephalus. The symptoms usually include paralysis, INCONTINENCE, a high risk of meningitis and mental retardation. There is usually an abnormally high level of ALPHA-FETOPROTEIN in the amniotic fluid, and since this can be diagnosed and then confirmed by AMNIOCENTESIS, it is possible to terminate these pregnancies.

spinal anaesthesia the generation of ANAESTHESIA by injecting anaesthetic into the cerebrospinal fluid around the spinal cord. Of the two types, the EPIDURAL involves injecting into the outer lining of the spinal cord, while subarachnoid anaesthesia is produced by injecting between vertebrae in the lumbar region of the vertebral column. Spinal anaesthesia is useful for patients who have a condition that precludes a general anaesthetic (e.g. a chest infection or HEART DISEASE).

sponge, contraceptive a soft sponge that is impregnated with SPERMICIDE and placed over the CERVIX, used as a means of CONTRACEPTION. It is easy to use but can have a failure rate of up to 25 per cent (75 per cent effective) so it is no longer available in the UK. It is still popular in the USA.

sterilization a surgical operation to render someone physically incapable of having children. In women, the operation may be carried out through the abdomen or the VAGINA. The procedure involves interrupting the connection between UTERUS and FALLOPIAN TUBES by TUBAL LIGATION, CAUTERIZATION and clips. A HYSTERECTOMY also produces sterilization. (*See also* TUBAL LIGATION).

stillbirth the birth of a child, after 28 weeks GESTATION, that has no evidence of life. The reasons include foetal defects, placental insufficiency, RHESUS INCOMPATIBILITY, ANAEMIA, INFECTION, UMBILICAL CORD problems, uncontrolled maternal DIABETES and ECLAMPSIA. (*See also* MISCARRIAGE; PREMATURE BIRTH).

stress any external or internal influence that has, or potentially has, an adverse effect on the correct functioning of the body. These influences include physical factors, such as disease or injury, or mental ones, particularly ANXIETY. Some degree of stress is necessary to keep people alert. Problems develop when a person can no longer handle the emotional, physical and mental stresses encountered in everyday life.

Symptoms such as FATIGUE, NAUSEA, indigestion, PALPITATIONS, INSOMNIA, anxiety, irritation, HEADACHES and chest pain may develop, as stress changes the hormonal balance in the body and lowers the effectiveness of the IMMUNE SYSTEM, leading to a higher risk of INFECTION. Changes in lifestyle, relaxation techniques and dealing with emotional difficulties can reduce mental stress and alleviate physical symptoms. Physical diseases and injuries can be treated and counselling offered to help patients deal with stress caused by pain and prolonged illness.

stress incontinence an involuntary release of URINE as a result of some action that increases abdominal pressure on the BLADDER, e.g. sneezing or coughing. It is caused by a weakening of the PELVIC FLOOR MUSCLES, especially the PUBOCOCCYGEOUS muscle, which can occur after childbirth. Mild stress incontinence can be helped by KEGEL EXERCISES to strengthen the muscles, but corrective surgery may be needed in more severe cases. (*See also* PROLAPSE; URETHROCELE; CYSTOCELE; RECTOCELE).

stretch marks (STRIAE gravidarum) pink streaks that develop on the abdomen, BREASTS, thighs or buttocks after WEIGHT GAIN or in late PREGNANCY. The skin loses its elasticity when the fibres are overstretched and in time the marks fade to a white, silvery colour.

striae fine lines or elongated bands or ribbons.

stroke the physical effects, involving some form of paralysis, that result from an interruption to the brain's BLOOD supply. The effect on the brain is secondary and is due to a THROMBUS, embolus or HAEMORRHAGE in the heart or blood vessels. The severity of a stroke can vary from temporary weakness of a limb to paralysis, coma and death.

superfecundation the FERTILIZATION of two EGGS during the same MENSTRUAL CYCLE but not during the same act of SEXUAL INTERCOURSE. This results in the CONCEPTION of fraternal (dizygotic) twins or other form of MULTIPLE PREGNANCY.

suppository medication prepared in a form that enables it to be inserted into the RECTUM. It may be a lubricant, drugs for treatment in the area of the rectum or anus, or for absorption into the boodstream. The suppository has to be inserted beyond the sphincter muscle to ensure retention.

syphilis an infectious, SEXUALLY TRANSMITTED DISEASE, caused by the bacterium *Treponema pallidum*, that shows symptoms in 3 stages. Bacteria enter the body through MUCOUS MEMBRANES during SEXUAL INTERCOURSE, and an ulcer appears in the first instance. Within a short time the LYMPH nodes locally, and then all over the body, enlarge and harden, and this lasts several weeks. Secondary symptoms appear about 2 months after INFECTION and include FEVER, pains, enlarged lymph nodes and a faint rash that is usually noticed on the chest. The bacteria are found in enormous numbers in the primary sores and any skin lesions of the secondary stage. The final stage may not appear until many months or years after infection and comprises the formation of numerous tumour-like masses throughout the body (in skin, muscle, BONE, brain, spinal cord and other organs such as the liver, stomach, etc). This stage can cause serious damage to the heart, brain or spinal cord, resulting in blindness and mental disability. Congenital syphilis is much rarer than the former, acquired, type. It is contracted by a developing FOETUS from the mother across the PLACENTA, and symptoms show a few weeks after birth. Treatment of syphilis is with penicillin, but it should be administered early in the development of the disease.

systemic lupus erythematosus (SLE) an AUTOIMMUNE DISEASE 90 per cent of the sufferers of which are women aged mainly between 30 and 50. It develops as a result of an allergic reaction to collagen in the arteries, which is destroyed. Damage occurs in the skin, kidneys, joints, heart and lungs, although in severe cases all tissues and organs are affected. Symptoms include swelling and pain in joints, chest pain and breathlessness, enlargement of GLANDS, kidney failure, and a characteristic skin rash ('butterfly') over the nose and cheeks. The disease is diagnosed by BLOOD TESTS for the antinuclear factor. It is usually CHRONIC with active phases and quiescent periods of REMISSION. In severe cases SLE can be life-threatening. Treatment is by anti-inflammatory drugs and immunosuppressants, with physiotherapy to help joint mobility. The pattern of development is variable, but renal failure, very high BLOOD PRESSURE and damage of the IMMUNE SYSTEM are extremely common. Ultraviolet light can accelerate the condition, which is more common in black people.

T

Tay-Sachs disease a fatal hereditary disorder of lipid METABOLISM in which abnormal accumulation of lipid in the brain leads to blindness, mental retardation and convulsions. It is caused by a recessive GENE that is 10 times more common in certain Central and Eastern European races. There is no cure, and GENETIC COUNSELLING can determine if a person is a carrier. AMNIOCENTESIS can detect the disorder in a FOETUS.

termination of pregnancy *see* ABORTION.

thalassaemia (Cooley's anaemia) an inherited form of ANAEMIA in which there is an abnormality in the HAEMOGLOBIN. There is a continuation in the production of foetal haemoglobin, and two forms of the disorder are recognized: T. major, in which the disorder is inherited from both parents (homozygous); and T. minor. The minor form is usually symptomless, but the major type causes, in addition to the severe anaemia, BONE MARROW abnormalities and enlargement of the spleen. Treatment is by means of repeated BLOOD transfusions. The disease is widespread throughout the Mediterranean, Asia and Africa.

thermography a method of recording the heat produced by different areas of the body, using photographic film sensitive to infrared radiation. Areas with good BLOOD circulation produce more heat, and this can occur abnormally if a tumour is present. The record thus obtained is a **thermogram,** and this is one of the techniques used to detect BREAST CANCER tumours.

thrombus a BLOOD CLOT within a vessel that partially or totally obstructs the circulation.

thrush a common vaginal INFECTION that causes severe ITCHING of the VAGINA and VULVA. There is normally a thick, white vaginal discharge that resembles cottage cheese. The infection is caused by a fungus, *Candida albicans*, that normally lives in the vagina where the acidic environment usually keeps it at low levels. Thrush develops only when the acidic balance in the vagina changes. This may be caused by taking some antibiotics, ORAL CONTRACEPTIVES or by raised levels of OESTROGEN in PREGNANCY. An increase in blood sugar can cause *Candida* to multiply, as can faecal contamination, tight-fitting clothes, an INTRAUTERINE DEVICE and some chemicals in soap, bath foam or detergents.

Thrush can be triggered by SEXUAL INTERCOURSE and may be transmitted between partners, although it causes few symptoms in men. The infection can be eased by eating live yoghurt (which suppresses the bacterial and fungal growth in the intestines) or using this as a vaginal application. A SITZ BATH with lemon juice or vinegar in the water is helpful. These all increase the acidity of the vagina, making it less hospitable to thrush. Conventional treatment consists of fungal antibiotics, as cream and/or vaginal pessaries, the most widely used of which is clotrimazole. It can be obtained from pharmacies without prescription. A recent study found that some recurrent attacks of thrush in certain women were connected to an allergic reaction to the partner's semen. This can be prevented by using a CONDOM and treated with a course of antihistamine tablets to stop the reaction. Thrush can also occur on the skin, in the intestinal tract and in the mouth. Oral infection with *Candida* is particularly prevalent in people with AIDS.

thyroid gland a bi-lobed ENDOCRINE GLAND situated at the base and front of the neck. It is enclosed by fibrous tissue and well supplied with BLOOD, and internally consists of numerous vesicles containing a jelly-like colloidal substance. These vesicles produce thyroid HORMONE, which is rich in iodine, under the control of thyroid-stimulating hormone (thyrotrophin-stimulating hormone) released from the PITUITARY GLAND. Two hormones are produced by the gland, thyroxine and triiodothyronine, which are essential for the regulation of METABOLISM and growth.

toxaemia of pregnancy *see* ECLAMPSIA; PRE-ECLAMPSIA.

toxic shock syndrome a state of ACUTE shock due to septicaemia and caused by toxins produced by *staphylococcal* bacteria. The symptoms include high FEVER, skin rash and DIARRHOEA, and can prove rapidly fatal if not adequately treated with antibiotics, especially penicillin and cephalosporin, along with fluid and salt replacement. The syndrome is associated with the use of tampons by women during MENSTRUATION. Young women or girls whose IMMUNE SYSTEM is not fully developed may be at greater risk, particularly if a tampon is left in place too long. However, the syndrome can also occur in other people and is in all cases rare.

toxoplasmosis an infectious disease caused by a protozoan organism known as *Toxoplasma*. The INFECTION is either transmitted by eating undercooked meat or through direct contact with contaminated soil or especially with infected cats. This form of the infection is mild and causes few ill-effects. However, a much more serious form of the disease can be passed from a mother infected during PREGNANCY to her unborn baby. The newborn infant may suffer from hydrocephalus, mental retardation, blindness or may even be stillborn. Treatment is by means of sulphonamide drugs and pyrimethamine.

tranquillizer a drug that has a soothing and calming effect, relieving STRESS and ANXIETY. Minor tranquillizers such as diazepam and chlordiazepoxide are widely used to relieve these symptoms, which may arise from a variety of causes. There is a danger of dependence with long-term use. Major tranquillizers, e.g. chlor-promazine and haloperidol, are used to treat severe mental illnesses such as SCHIZO-PHRENIA.

trichomonas a vaginal INFECTION, caused by *Trichomonas vaginalis* (a protozoal microorganism), that is common in sexually active women. Symptoms include a yellow/green frothy discharge, itching of the VAGINA and VULVA, and CYSTITIS if the BLADDER is affected. Treatment is by means of metidazole, which cannot be used in PREGNANCY. All partners need to be treated, as *Trichomonas* can be spread by sexual contact.

trimester a three-month period, particularly those of PREGNANCY.

tubal ligation a surgical closing of the FALLOPIAN TUBES in order to prevent PREGNANCY. It is the main form of female STERILIZATION and can be carried out through an abdominal or vaginal incision. The tubes are clipped, cauterized or severed by laser to stop the passage of SPERM or EGGS. The procedure is normally irreversible and should be carried out only if a woman is certain she does not wish to have more children. Tubal ligation fails occasionally, usually because of incomplete closing of the tubes.

tuboplasty a surgical repair of FALLOPIAN TUBES in order to remove a blockage caused by scar tissue or to reverse TUBAL LIGATION. The success of the operation depends on the extent of scar tissue and the reason it formed or on the type of ligation carried out.

Turner's syndrome a genetic disorder affecting females in which there is only one X-CHROMOSOME instead of the usual two. Hence, those affected have 45 instead of 46 CHROMOSOMES, are infertile (as the ovaries are not present), MENSTRUATION is absent and BREASTS and body hair do not develop. Those affected are short, may have webbing of the neck and other developmental defects. The heart may be affected, and there can be deafness and intellectual impairment. In a less severe form, the second X-chromosome is present but abnormal, lacking in normal genetic material.

turning *see* VERSION.

U

ultrasound high frequency sound waves (above 20 kHz), beyond the range of the human ear. Ultrasound is used to examine the body's organs, ducts, etc, in addition to assessing the progress of a developing FOETUS. The patient is not submitted to harmful radiation, as with other techniques, and no contrast medium is required. It can be used to examine the liver, kidney, BLADDER, PANCREAS and ovaries, and is used in diagnosing brain tumours. The vibrations of the sound waves can be used in other ways, e.g. breaking up kidney stones. The technique can detect OVARIAN CYSTS, ECTOPIC PREGNANCY, GALLSTONES, hernias and abnormality in BREAST tissue in younger women.

umbilical vein sampling under the guidance of ULTRASOUND, a small sample of BLOOD is removed from a blood vessel in the UMBILICAL CORD *in utero*. This can be tested to detect INFECTIONS like GERMAN MEASLES, HERPES and TOXOPLASMOSIS, and to check the CHROMOSOME count or effects on the FOETUS of RHESUS INCOMPATIBILITY. Suspected growth retardation can also be investigated. The risk of miscarriage may be 1–2 per cent. (*See also* AMNIOCENTESIS; CHORIONIC VILLUS SAMPLING).

umbilical cord the cord connecting the FOETUS to the PLACENTA, containing two arteries and one VEIN. It is approximately 60 cm long, and after birth it is severed and the stump shrivels to leave a scar, the navel or umbilicus.

ureaplasma or **urealyticum** one of a group of Ureplasma microorganisms that causes INFLAMMATION of the ENDOMETRIUM (and prostate gland in males) and nonspecific URETHRITIS. The organisms are commonly present in the urinary and genital tract, and may be transferred through SEXUAL INTERCOURSE. INFECTION can lead to early MISCARRIAGE (and foetal death) and the formation of ANTIBODIES against SPERM, leading to INFERTILITY, and may cause CERVICITIS in some women.

urethra the duct carrying URINE from the BLADDER out of the body. It is about 3.5 cm long in women and 20 cm in men. Problems with bladder control can develop after childbirth or the MENOPAUSE, and this can lead to STRESS INCONTINENCE. URETHRITIS is a common problem in women and is often accompanied by bladder infections such as CYSTITIS.

urethritis INFLAMMATION of the mucous lining of the URETHRA that may be associated with CYSTITIS, often being the cause of the latter. The commonest cause of urethritis is GONORRHOEA (specific urethritis). Alternatively, it may be caused by INFECTION with microorganisms (nonspecific urethritis). The symptoms include a discharge, pain on passing URINE, and inflammation in other organs, such as the BLADDER, is possible. Sulphonamide and antibiotic drugs are effective, once the infecting organism is identified.

urethrocele protrusion of the URETHRA into the VAGINA because of weak PELVIC FLOOR MUSCLES. It generally occurs with CYSTOCELE and is treated in the same way.

urine the body's fluid waste excreted by the kidneys. The waste products include urea, uric acid and creatinine (produced by muscles), with salt, phosphates and sulphates and ammonia also present. In a solution with about 95–96 per cent water, there may be 100 or more compounds, but the vast majority occur only in trace amounts. Many diseases alter the quantity and composition of urine, and its analysis is standard procedure to assist DIAGNOSIS.

urine test laboratory analysis to detect BLOOD, sugar, protein or bacteria that may be present in URINE. HORMONE levels in a woman can be determined by analysis of urine samples over a 24-hour period.

uterine cancer a MALIGNANT growth of abnormal cells in the UTERUS or womb. (*See also* CERVICAL CANCER; ENDOMETRIAL CANCER.)

uterine polyp *see* POLYP.

uterus a vaguely pear-shaped organ within the cavity of the PELVIS that is specialized for the growth and nourishment of a FOETUS. FALLOPIAN TUBES connect to the upper part, and the lower end joins the VAGINA at the CERVIX. It has a plentiful BLOOD supply with LYMPHatic vessels and nerves. During PREGNANCY it enlarges considerably and the smooth muscle walls thicken. CONTRACTIONS of the muscular wall push the foetus out via the vagina at childbirth. If there is no pregnancy, the lining undergoes periodic changes (MENSTRUATION). The uterus is subject to numerous disorders, including FIBROIDS, POLYPS, PELVIC INFLAMMATORY DISEASE, UTERINE CANCER and PROLAPSE. Removal of the uterus (HYSTERECTOMY) and scraping of the uterine lining (D AND C) are two of the most common surgical procedures in women.

V

vacuum aspiration a method of removing tissue from the UTERUS, which can be used to obtain samples of the ENDOMETRIUM or to remove placental and foetal tissue in a first trimester ABORTION.

vagina the lower part of the female reproductive tract that leads from the UTERUS to the exterior. It receives the erect penis during SEXUAL INTERCOURSE. The semen is ejaculated into the upper part, from where the sperm pass through the CERVIX and UTERUS to the FALLO-PIAN TUBES. The vagina is a muscular tube lined with MUCOUS MEM-BRANE. It is subject to several conditions, including THRUSH, TRICHOMONAS, VAGINITIS and VAGINAL CANCER.

vaginal atrophy loss of elasticity with dryness and thinning of the tissues that line the vaginal walls (also including the UTERUS, VULVA and URETHRA). This develops after the MENOPAUSE, when lower levels of OESTROGEN result in a fall in mucus production. The use of lubricants can help the condition, as can HORMONE REPLACEMENT THERAPY. There may be pain during intercourse and higher risks of urethral, urinary and vaginal INFLAMMATION and INFECTION.

vaginal cancer abnormal growth of MALIGNANT cells in vaginal tissues. It is a rare CANCER except in daughters of women who took DES (diethylstilboesterol) in PREGNANCY. These women have abnormal glandular tissue in the VAGINA, which can give rise to an unusual form of adenocarcinoma. Vaginal cancer may be treated with surgery and/or RADIOTHERAPY.

vaginismus a sudden and painful contraction of muscles surrounding the VAGINA in response to contact of the vagina or VULVA, e.g. attempted intercourse. It may be caused by a fear of intercourse or an INFLAMMATION.

vaginitis INFLAMMATION of the VAGINA that produces severe ITCHING and burning of the VULVA and often a vaginal discharge. This can be due to INFECTION, poor HYGIENE or dietary deficiency. Hormonal changes can allow development of an infection, the most common being THRUSH, but also TRICHOMONAS, HERPES, GONORRHOEA, CYSTS, CHLAMYDIA, etc. Treatment includes antibiotics and other drugs, strict hygiene, and wearing loose clothing and natural fibres so as not to create an environment favourable to infective organisms.

varicose veins VEINS that have become stretched, distended and twisted. The superficial veins in the legs are often affected, although it may occur elsewhere. Causes include congenitally defective valves, OBESITY, PREGNANCY and also thrombophlebitis (INFLAMMATION of the wall of a vein with secondary thrombosis in the affected part). Elastic support is a common treatment, although others include sclerotherapy and phlebotomy (surgical removal of a vein).

vein one of the numerous BLOOD vessels carrying deoxygenated blood to the right atrium of the heart (the one exception is the pulmonary vein). Each vein has three tissue layers, similar to the layers of the heart. Veins are less elastic than arteries and collapse when cut. They also contain valves to prevent backflow.

ventouse delivery a method of assisted DELIVERY that uses a suction cup attached to the head by a vacuum to pull the baby gently through the BIRTH CANAL. It is used as an alternative to FORCEPS when there is a delay in the second stage of LABOUR. This method results in little damage and is more popular in Europe.

version or **turning** the procedure to move a FOETUS in the UTERUS to a more normal position to make DELIVERY easier.

virus the smallest microbe that is completely parasitic, because it is capable of replication only within the cells of its host. Viruses infect animals, plants and microorganisms. They are classified according to their NUCLEIC ACIDS and can contain double or single-stranded DNA or RNA. In an INFECTION the virus binds to the host cells and then penetrates the cell membrane to release its DNA or RNA, which controls the cell's METABOLISM and enables it to replicate itself and form new viruses. Viruses cause many diseases, including influenza (single-stranded RNA), HERPES (double-stranded DNA), AIDS (a retrovirus, single-stranded RNA) and also mumps, chickenpox and polio.

vitamin any of a group of organic compounds required in very small amounts in the diet to maintain good health. Deficiencies lead to specific diseases. Vitamins are divided into 2 groups: vitamins A, D, E and K are fat-soluble, while C and B are water soluble.

vomiting the reflex action whereby the stomach contents are expelled through the mouth because of the contraction of the DIAPHRAGM and abdominal wall muscles. Vomiting is due to stimulus of the appropriate centre in the brain, but the primary agent is usually a sensation from the stomach itself, e.g. a gastric disease or some irritant. Other causes may be the action of drugs, some effect on the inner ear (e.g. travel sickness), MIGRAINE, etc.

vulva the external genitalia in women that include the MONS VENERIS, LABIA majora and labia minora, CLITORIS and the opening to the

VAGINA. This area is liable to conditions such as SEXUALLY TRANS-MITTED DISEASES, VULVAR CANCER and VULVITIS.

vulvar cancer a form of SKIN CANCER in which a MALIGNANT lump or sore grows in the VULVA. It is more common after the MENOPAUSE, and while it can usually be seen and felt, many women fail to seek treatment because of embarrassment. The LESION resembles those found in GENITAL HERPES, and a BIOPSY is needed to distinguish the two conditions. Rarely, a malignant melanoma may develop on the vulva. Treatment is by means of surgery, which may need to be quite extensive, and RADIOTHERAPY.

vulvitis INFLAMMATION of the VULVA that can be caused by PUBIC LICE, HERPES or a vaginal INFECTION. Contact with some detergents, bubble bath or CONDOMS can cause allergic dermatitis. Allergic reaction to some drugs or antibiotics can result in vulvitis. Treatment is by SITZ BATHS or compresses, to relieve inflammation and ITCHING, and various creams and preparations. LESIONS or discharge require investigation for DIAGNOSIS of infection or malignancy.

W

wart a solid, BENIGN growth in the skin caused by a VIRUS. They are infectious and spread rapidly in schools, etc. There are several types: plantar, on the foot; juvenile in children; and venereal, on the GENITALS. Warts often disappear spontaneously but can be dealt with in several ways, e.g. CRYOSURGERY, laser treatment and electrocautery (burning away with an electrically heated wire or needle). (*See also* GENITAL HERPES.)

weight, body the actual body weight, which varies somewhat throughout adult life. Advisable weight is dependent on height and general body frame. WEIGHT GAIN is a common problem in much of the industrialized world, but weight loss can indicate several disorders. (*See also* ANOREXIA NERVOSA; BIRTH WEIGHT; CRITICAL WEIGHT; NUTRITION; OBESITY.)

weight gain many women gain weight in the week before the MENSTRUAL CYCLE, usually because of FLUID RETENTION and increased appetite. Weight gain after the MENOPAUSE is quite common because the METABOLISM slows down. This increases the risk of ARTERIO-SCLEROSIS, HEART DISEASE, HYPERTENSION and DIABETES. During PREG-NANCY a weight gain of 24–28 pounds is normal but varies considerably. Weight gain can be a symptom of many disorders, including hormonal and THYROID GLAND disturbance.

womb the common name for the UTERUS.

XYZ

X chromosome the sex CHROMOSOME present in males and females, although women have a pair and men just one (with one Y-CHRO-MOSOME). Certain disorders such as HAEMOPHILIA are carried as GENES on the X chromosome.

X-rays the part of the electromagnetic spectrum with waves of wavelength 10–12 to 10–9m and frequencies of 1017–1021Hz. They are produced when high velocity electrons strike a target. The rays penetrate solids to a depth that depends on the density of the solid. X-rays of certain wavelengths will penetrate flesh but not BONE. They are therefore useful in therapy and DIAGNOSIS within medicine.

Y-chromosome the small CHROMOSOME that carries a dominant GENE conferring maleness. Normal males have 22 matched chromosome pairs and one unmatched pair, comprising one X-CHROMOSOME and one Y-chromosome. During sexual reproduction the mother contributes an X CHROMOSOME, but the father contributes an X- or Y-chromosome. XX produces a female offspring, XY a male.

zygote the cell produced by the fusion of male and female germ cells (GAMETES) during the early stage of FERTILIZATION, i.e. an OVUM fertilized by a SPERM. After passing down the FALLOPIAN TUBE, it implants in the UTERUS, forming the EMBRYO.

Guide to Popular
Complementary Therapies

Acupressure

This is an ancient form of healing combining massage and acupuncture, practised over 3,000 years ago in Japan and China. It was developed into its current form using a system of special massage points and is today still practised widely in the Japanese home environment. Certain 'pressure points' are located in various parts of the body and these are used by the practitioner by massaging firmly with the thumb or fingertip. These points are the same as those utilized in acupuncture. There are various ways of working and the pressure can be applied by the practitioner's fingers, thumbs, knees, palms of the hand, etc. Relief from pain can be quite rapid at times, depending upon its cause, while other more persistent problems can take longer to improve.

Acupressure is said to enhance the body's own method of healing, thereby preventing illness and improving the energy level. The pressure exerted is believed to regulate a matter called 'Qi', which is energy that flows along 'meridians'. These are invisible channels that run along the length of the body. These meridians are mainly named after the organs of the body such as the liver and stomach, but there are four exceptions, which are called the 'pericardium', 'triple heater', 'conception' and 'governor'. Specifically named meridian lines may also be used to treat ailments other than those relating to it.

Ailments claimed to have been treated successfully are back pain, asthma, digestive problems, insomnia, migraine and circulatory problems, amongst others. Changes in diet, regular exercise and certain self-checking methods may be recommended by your practitioner. It must be borne in mind that some painful symptoms are the onset of serious illness so you should always first consult your G.P.

Before any treatment commences, a patient will be asked details of lifestyle and diet, the pulse rate will be taken along with any relevant past history relating to the current problem. The person will be requested to lie on a mattress on the floor or on a firm table, and comfortable but loose-fitting clothing is best so that the practitioner can work most effectively on the energy channels. No oils are used on the body and there is no equipment. Each session lasts from approximately 30 minutes to 1 hour. Once the pressure is applied, and this can be done in a variety of ways particular to each practitioner, varying sensations may be felt. Some points may feel sore or tender and there may be some discomfort such as a deep pain or coolness. However, it is believed that this form of massage works quickly so that any tenderness soon passes.

The number of treatments will vary from patient to patient, according to how the person responds and what problem or ailment is being treated. Weekly visits may be needed if a specific disorder is being treated while other people may go whenever they feel in need. It is advisable for women who are pregnant to check with their practitioner first since some of the acupressure methods are not recommended during pregnancy. Acupressure can be practised safely at home although it is usually better for one person to perform the massage on another. Common problems such as headache, constipation and toothache can be treated quite simply although there is the possibility of any problem worsening first before an improvement occurs if the pressure points are over stimulated. You should, however, see your doctor if any ailment persists. To treat headache, facial soreness, toothache and menstrual pain, locate the fleshy piece of skin between the thumb and forefinger and squeeze firmly, pressing towards the forefinger. The pressure should be applied for about five minutes and either hand can be used. This point is known as 'Large Intestine 4'.

To aid digestive problems in both adults and babies, for example to settle infantile colic, the point known as 'Stomach 36' is utilized, which is located on the outer side of the leg about 75mm (3ins) down from the knee. This point should be quite simple to find as it can often feel slightly tender. It should be pressed quite firmly and strongly for about five to ten minutes with the thumb.

When practising acupressure massage on someone else and before treatment begins, ensure that the person is warm, relaxed, comfortable and wearing loose-fitting clothing and that he or she is lying on a firm mattress or rug on the floor. To discover the areas that need to be worked on, press firmly over the body and see which areas are tender. These tender areas on the body correspond to an organ that is not working correctly. To commence massage using fingertips or thumbs, a pressure of about 4.5 kg (10 lbs) should be exerted. The massage movements should be performed very quickly, about 50 to 100 times every minute, and some discomfort is likely (which will soon pass) but there should be no pain. Particular care should be taken to avoid causing pain on the face, stomach or over any joints. If a baby or young child is being massaged then considerably less pressure should be used. If there is any doubt as to the correct amount, exert a downwards pressure on bathroom scales to ascertain the weight being used. There is no need to hurry from one point to another since approximately 5 to 15 minutes is needed at each point for adults, but only about 30 seconds for babies or young children.

Using the 'self-help' acupressure, massage can be repeated as often as is felt to be necessary with several sessions per hour usually being sufficient for painful conditions that have arisen suddenly. It is possible that as many as 20 sessions may be necessary for persistent conditions causing pain, with greater intervals of time between treatments as matters improve. It is not advisable to try anything that is at all complicated (or to treat an illness such as arthritis) and a trained practitioner will obviously be able to provide the best level of treatment and help. To contact a reputable practitioner who has completed the relevant training it is advisable to contact the appropriate professional body.

Acupuncture

This is an ancient Chinese therapy that involves inserting needles into the skin at specific points of the body. The word 'acupuncture' originated from a Dutch physician, William Ten Rhyne, who had been living in Japan during the latter part of the 17th century and it was he who introduced it to Europe. The term means literally 'prick with a needle'. The earliest textbook on acupuncture, dating from approximately 400 BC, was called *Nei Ching Su Wen*, which means 'Yellow Emperor's Classic of Internal Medicine'. Also recorded at about the same time was the successful saving of a patient's life by acupuncture, the person having been expected to die whilst in a coma. Legend has it that acupuncture was developed when it was realized that soldiers who recovered from arrow wounds were sometimes also healed of other diseases from which they were suffering. Acupuncture was very popular with British doctors in the early 1800s for pain relief and to treat fever. There was also a specific article on the successful treatment of rheumatism that appeared in *The Lancet*. Until the end of the Ching dynasty in China in 1911, acupuncture was slowly developed and improved, but then medicine from the West increased in popularity. However, more recently there has been a revival of interest and it is again widely practised throughout China. Also, nowadays the use of laser beams and electrical currents are found to give an increased stimulative effect when using acupuncture needles.

The specific points of the body into which acupuncture needles are inserted are located along 'meridians'. These are the pathways or energy channels and are believed to be related to the internal organs of the body. This energy is known as *qi* and the needles are used to decrease or increase the flow of energy, or to unblock it if it is impeded. Traditional Chinese medicine sees the body as being comprised of two natural forces known as the *yin* and *yang*. These two forces are complementary to each other but also opposing, the yin being the female force and calm and passive and also representing the dark, cold, swelling and moisture. The yang force is the male and is stimulating and aggressive, representing the heat and light, contraction and dryness. It is believed that the cause of ailments and diseases is due to an imbalance of these forces in the body, e.g. if a person is suffering from a headache or high blood pressure then this is because of an excess of yang. If, however, there is an excess of yin, this might result in tiredness, feeling cold and fluid retention .

The aim of acupuncture is to establish that there is an imbalance of yin and yang and to rectify it by using the needles at certain points on the body. Traditionally there were 365 points but more have been found in the intervening period and nowadays there can be as many as 2,000. There are 14 meridians, called after the organs they represent, e.g. the lung, kidney, heart and stomach as well as two organs unknown in orthodox medicine—the triple heater or warmer, which relates to the activity of the endocrine glands and the control of temperature. In addition, the pericardium is concerned with seasonal activity and also regulates the circulation of the blood. Of the 14 meridians, there are two, known as the *du,* or governor, and the *ren*, or conception, which both run straight up the body's midline, although the du is much shorter, extending from the head down to the mouth, while the ren starts at the chin and extends to the base of the trunk.

There are several factors that can change the flow of qi (also known as shi or ch'i), and they can be of an emotional, physical or environmental nature. The flow may be changed to become too slow or fast, or it can be diverted or blocked so that the incorrect organ is involved and the acupuncturist has to ensure that the flow returns to normal. There are many painful afflictions for which acupuncture can be used. In the West, it has been used primarily for rheumatism, back pain and arthritis, but it has also been used to alleviate other disorders such as stress, allergy, colitis, digestive troubles, insomnia, asthma, etc. It has been claimed that withdrawal symptoms (experienced by people stopping smoking and ceasing other forms of addiction) have been helped as well.

Qualified acupuncturists complete a training course of three years duration and also need qualifications in the related disciplines of anatomy, pathology, physiology and diagnosis before they can belong to a professional association. It is very important that a fully qualified acupuncturist, who is a member of the relevant professional body, is consulted because at the present time, any unqualified person can use the title 'acupuncturist'.

At a consultation, the traditional acupuncturist uses a set method of ancient rules to determine the acupuncture points. The texture and colouring of the skin, type of skin, posture and movement and the tongue will all be examined and noted, as will the patient's voice. These different factors are all needed for the Chinese diagnosis. A number of questions will be asked concerning the diet, amount of exercise taken, lifestyle, fears and phobias, sleeping patterns and reactions to stress. Each wrist has six pulses, and each of these stand for a main organ and its function. The pulses are felt (known as palpating), and by this means acupuncturists are able to diagnose any problems relating to the flow of qi and if there is any disease present in the internal organs. The first consultation may last an hour, especially if detailed questioning is necessary along with the palpation.

The needles used in acupuncture are disposable and made of a fine stainless steel and come already sealed in a sterile pack. They can be sterilized by the acupuncturist in a machine known as an autoclave but using boiling water is not adequate for this purpose. (Diseases such as HIV and hepatitis can be passed on by using unsterilized needles.) Once the needle is inserted into the skin it is twisted between the acupuncturist's thumb and forefinger to spread or draw the energy from a point. The depth to which the needle is inserted can vary from just below the skin to up to 12mm (half an inch) and different sensations may be felt, such as a tingling around the area of insertion or a loss of sensation at that point. Up to 15 needles can be used but around five is generally sufficient. The length of time that they are left in varies from a few minutes to half an hour and this is dependent on a number of factors such as how the patient has reacted to previous treatment and the ailment from which he or she is suffering.

Patients can generally expect to feel an improvement after four to six sessions of therapy, the beneficial effects occurring gradually, particularly if the ailment has obvious and long-standing symptoms.

Other diseases such as asthma will probably take longer before any definite improvement is felt. It is possible that some patients may not feel any improvement at all, or even feel worse after the first session and this is probably due to the energies in the body being over-stimulated. To correct this, the acupuncturist will gradually use fewer needles and for a shorter period of time. If no improvement is felt after about six to eight treatments, then it is doubtful whether acupuncture will be of any help. For general body maintenance and health, most traditional acupuncturists suggest that sessions be arranged at the time of seasonal changes.

There has been a great deal of research, particularly by the Chinese, who have produced many books detailing a high success rate for acupuncture in treating a variety of disorders. These results are, however, viewed cautiously in the West as methods of conducting clinical trials vary from East to West. Nevertheless trials have been carried out in the West and it has been discovered that a pain message can be stopped from reaching the brain using acupuncture. The signal would normally travel along a nerve but it is possible to 'close a gate' on the nerve, thereby preventing the message from reaching the brain, hence preventing the perception of pain. Acupuncture is believed to work by blocking the pain signal. However, doctors stress that pain can be a warning that something is wrong or of the occurrence of a particular disease, such as cancer, that requires an orthodox remedy or method of treatment.

It has also been discovered that there are substances, called endorphins and encephalins, produced by the body that are connected with pain relief. Studies from all over the world show that acupuncture stimulates the release of these opiates into the central nervous system, thereby giving pain relief. The amount of opiates released has a direct bearing on the degree of pain relief. Acupuncture is a widely used form of anaesthesia in China where, for suitable patients, it is said to be extremely effective (90 per cent). It is used successfully during childbirth, dentistry and for operations. Orthodox doctors in the West now accept that heat treatment, massage and needles used on a sensitive part of the skin afford relief from pain caused by disease elsewhere. These areas are known as trigger points, and they are not always situated close to the organ that is affected by disease. It has been found that approximately three-quarters of these trigger points are the same as the points used in Chinese acupuncture. Recent research has also shown that it is possible to find the acupuncture points by the use of electronic instruments as they register less electrical resistance than other areas of skin. As yet, no evidence has been found to substantiate the existence of meridians.

The Alexander Technique

This technique, which is based on correct posture so that the body is able to function naturally and with the minimum amount of muscular effort, was devised by Frederick Mathias Alexander (1869–1955). He was an Australian actor who found that he was losing his voice when performing but after rest his condition improved. Although he received medical help, the condition did not improve and it occurred to him that whilst acting he might be doing something that caused the problem. To see what this might be he performed his act in front of a mirror and saw what happened when he was about to speak. He experienced difficulty in breathing and lowered his head, thus making himself shorter. He realized that the strain of remembering his lines and having to project his voice, so that people furthest away in the audience would be able to hear, was causing him a great deal of stress and the way he reacted was a quite natural reflex action. In fact, even thinking about having to project his voice made the symptoms recur and from this he concluded that there must be a close connection between body and mind. He was determined to try and improve the situation and gradually, by watching and altering his stance and posture and his mental attitude to his performance on stage, matters improved. He was able to act and speak on stage and use his body in a more relaxed and natural fashion.

In 1904 Alexander travelled to London where he had decided to let others know about his method of retraining the body. He soon became very popular with other actors who appreciated the benefits of using his technique. Other public figures, such as the author Aldous Huxley, also benefited. Later he went to America, achieving considerable success and international recognition for his technique. At the age of 78 he suffered a stroke but by using his method he managed to regain the use of all his faculties—an achievement that amazed his doctors.

The Alexander technique is said to be completely harmless, encouraging an agreeable state between mind and body and is also helpful for a number of disorders such as headaches and back pain. Today, Alexander training schools can be found all over the world. A simple test to determine if people can benefit is to observe their posture. People frequently do not even stand correctly and this can encourage aches and pains if the body is unbalanced. It is incorrect to stand with round shoulders or to slouch. This often looks uncomfortable and discomfort may be felt. Sometimes people will hold themselves too erect and unbending, which again can have a bad effect. The correct posture and balance for the body needs the least muscular effort but the body will be aligned correctly. When walking one should not slouch, hold the head down or have the shoulders stooped. The head should be balanced correctly above the spine with the shoulders relaxed. It is suggested that the weight of the body should be felt being transferred from one foot to the other whilst walking.

Once a teacher has been consulted, all movements and how the body is used will be observed. Many muscles are used in everyday activities, and over the years bad habits can develop unconsciously, with stress also affecting the use of muscles. This can be demonstrated in people gripping a pen with too much force or holding the steering wheel of a car too tightly whilst driving. Muscular tension can be a serious problem affecting some people and the head, neck and back are forced out of line, which in turn leads to rounded shoulders with the head held forward and the back curved. If this situation is not altered and the body is not re-aligned correctly, the spine will become curved with a hump possibly developing. This leads to back pain and puts a strain on internal organs such as the chest and lungs.

No force is used by the teacher other than some gentle manipulation to start pupils off correctly. Some teachers use light pushing methods on the back and hips, etc, while others might first ensure that the pupil is relaxed and then pull gently on the neck, which stretches the body. Any bad postures will be corrected by the teacher and the pupil will be shown how best to alter this so that muscles will be used most effectively and with the least effort. Any manipulation that is used will be to ease the body into a more relaxed and natural position. It is helpful to be completely aware of using the technique not only on the body but also with the mind. With frequent use of the Alexander technique for posture and the release of tension, the muscles and the body should be used correctly with a consequent improvement in, for example, the manner of walking and sitting.

The length of time for each lesson can vary from about half an hour to three quarters of an hour and the number of lessons is usually between 10 and 30, by which time pupils should have gained sufficient knowledge to continue practising the technique by themselves. Once a person has learned how to improve posture, it will be found that he or she is taller and carrying the body in a more upright manner. The technique has been found to be of benefit to dancers, athletes and those having to speak in public. Other disorders claimed to have been treated successfully are depressive states, headaches caused by tension, anxiety, asthma, hypertension, respiratory problems, colitis, osteoarthritis and rheumatoid arthritis, sciatica and peptic ulcer.

The Alexander technique is recommended for all ages and types of people as their overall quality of life, both mental and physical, can be improved. People can learn how to resist stress and one eminent professor experienced a great improvement in a variety of ways: in quality of sleep; lessening of high blood pressure and improved mental awareness. He even found that his ability to play a musical instrument had improved.

The Alexander technique can be applied to two positions adopted every day, namely sitting in a chair and sitting at a desk. To be seated in the correct manner the head should be comfortably balanced, with no tension in the shoulders, and a small gap between the knees (if legs are crossed the spine and pelvis become out of line or twisted) and the soles of the feet should be flat on the floor. It is incorrect to sit with the head lowered and the shoulders slumped forward because the stomach becomes restricted and breathing may also be affected. On the other hand, it is also incorrect to hold the body in a stiff and erect position.

To sit correctly while working at a table, the body should be held upright but in a relaxed manner with any bending movement coming from the hips and with the seat flat on the chair. If writing, the pen should be held lightly and if using a computer one should ensure that the arms are relaxed and feel comfortable. The chair should be set at a comfortable height with regard to the level of the desk. It is incorrect to lean forward over a desk because this hampers breathing, or to hold the arms in a tense, tight manner.

There has been some scientific research carried out that concurs with the beliefs that Alexander formed, such as the relationship between mind and body (the thought of doing an action actually triggering a physical reaction or tension). Today, doctors do not have any opposition to the Alexander technique and may recommend it on occasions.

Aromatherapy

Aromatherapy is a method of healing using very concentrated essential oils that are often highly aromatic and are extracted from plants. Constituents of the oils confer the characteristic perfume or odour given off by a particular plant. Essential oils help the plant in some way to complete its cycle of growth and reproduction. For example, some oils may attract insects for the purpose of pollination; others may render it distasteful as a source of food. Any part of a plant—the stems, leaves, flowers, fruits, seeds, roots or bark—may produce essential oils or essences but often only in minute amounts. Different parts of the same plant may produce their own form of oil. An example of this is the orange, which produces oils with different properties in the flowers, fruits and leaves.

The therapeutic and medicinal properties of plant extracts have long been recognized and their use dates back to earliest times. Art and writings from the ancient civilizations of Egypt, China and Persia show that plant essences were used and valued by priests, physicians and healers. Plant essences have been used throughout the ages for healing—in incense for religious rituals, in perfumes and embalming ointments and for culinary purposes. There are many Biblical references that give an insight into the uses of plant oils and the high value that was attached to them. Throughout the course of human history the healing properties of plants and their essential oils has been recognized and most people probably had some knowledge about their use. It was only in more recent times, with the great developments in science and orthodox medicine, particularly the manufacture of antibiotics and synthetic drugs, that knowledge and interest in the older methods of healing declined. However, in the last few years there has been a great rekindling of interest in the practice of aromatherapy with many people turning to this form of treatment.

Extraction of essential oils

Since any part of a plant may produce essential oils, the method of extraction depends upon the site and accessibility of the essence in each particular case. The oils are produced by special minute cells or glands and are released naturally by the plant in small amounts over a prolonged period of time when needed. In order to harvest the oils in appreciable amounts, it is usually necessary to collect a large quantity of the part of the plant needed and to subject the material to a process that causes the oil glands to burst. One of the most common methods is *steam distillation*. The plant material is paced tightly into a press or still and steamed at a high temperature. This causes the oil glands to burst and the essential oil vaporises into the steam. This is then cooled to separate the oil from the water. Sometimes water is used for distillation rather than steam. Another method involved dissolving the plant material in a solvent or alcohol and is called *solvent extraction*. This involves placing the material in a centrifuge, which rotates at high speed, and then extracting the essential oils by means of a low temperature distillation process. Substances obtained in this way may be called *resins* or *absolutes*. A further method is called *maceration* in which the plant is soaked in hot oil. The plant cells collapse and release their essential oils, and the whole mixture is then separated and purified by a process called *defleurage*. If fat is used instead of oil, the process is called *enfleurage*. These methods produce a purer oil that is usually more expensive than one obtained by distillation. The essential oils used in aromatherapy tend to be costly as vast quantities of plant material are required to produce them and the methods used are complex and costly.

Storage and use of essential oils

Essential oils are highly concentrated, volatile and aromatic. They readily evaporate and change and deteriorate if exposed to light, heat and air. Hence pure oils need to be stored carefully in brown glass bottles at a moderate temperature away from direct light. They can be stored for one or two years in this way. For most purposes in aromatherapy, essential oils are used in a dilute form, being added either to water or to another oil, called the *base* or *carrier*. The base is often a vegetable oil such as olive or safflower, which iboth have nutrient and beneficial properties. An essential/carrier oil mixture has a short useful life of two or three months and so they are usually mixed at the time of use and in small amounts.

Techniques used in aromatherapy

There are four techniques used in aromatherapy and these are *massage*, *bathing*, *inhalation* and *compresses*.

Massage is the most familiar method of treatment associated with aromatherapy. Essential oils are able to penetrate through the skin and are taken into the body, exerting healing and beneficial influences on internal tissues and organs. The oils used for massage are first diluted by being mixed with a base and should never be applied directly to the skin in their pure form in case of an adverse allergic reaction.

Bathing most people have experienced the benefits of relaxing in a hot bath to which a proprietary perfumed preparation has been added. Most of these preparations contain essential oils used in aromatherapy. The addition of a number of drops of an essential oil to the bath water can have great beneficial effects. It is soothing and relaxing, easing aches and pains, and can also have a stimulating effect, banishing tiredness and restoring energy, depending upon the type of oil that is used. In addition, there is the added benefit of inhaling the vapours of the oil as they evaporate from the hot water.

Inhalation isthought to be the most direct and rapid means of treatment. This is because the molecules of the volatile essential oil act directly on the olfactory organs and are immediately perceived by the brain. A popular method is the time-honoured one of *steam inhalation,* in which a few drops of essential oil are added to hot water in a bowl. The person sits with his or her face above the mixture and covers the head, face and bowl with a towel so that the vapours do not escape. This can be repeated up to three times a day but should not be undertaken by people suffering from asthma. Some essential oils can

be applied directly to a handkerchief or onto a pillow and the vapours inhaled in this way.

Compresses to prepare a compress in aromatherapy, a few drops of
essential oil are added to a proportion of hot or cold water and then
a cloth is soaked in the mixture. The cloth is wrung out, (although
kept fairly wet) and applied to the painful part, and is tied in place
with clingfilm and a bandage. The compress needs to be left in place
for two hours before being changed. Usually, hot compresses are applied to chronic persistent pain. For conditions in which there is heat,
inflammation, swelling and fever, a cold compress is generally indicated.

Essential oils may also be diluted with water and used in hand and
foot baths if only a small area of the body needs to be treated. Some
are appropriate for use as gargles and mouth washes, and are helpful
in clearing up infections such as mouth ulcers. However, they should
never be swallowed. Essential oils can be used effectively in the home
by adding a few drops into a bowl of water or potpourri and leaving
to stand in a room.

Mode of action of essential oils

Although the subject of a great deal of research, there is a lack of
knowledge about how essential oils work in the body to produce their
therapeutic effects. It is known that individual essential oils possess
antiseptic, antibiotic, sedative, tonic and stimulating properties, and
it is believed that they act in harmony with the natural defences of
the body such as the immune system. Some oils, such as eucalyptus
and rosemary, act as natural decongestants whereas others, such as
sage, have a beneficial effect upon the circulation.

Conditions that may benefit from aromatherapy

A wide range of conditions and disorders may benefit from
aromatherapy and it is considered to be a gentle treatment suitable
for all age groups. It is especially beneficial for long-term chronic con-

ditions, and the use of essential oils is believed by therapists to prevent the development of some illnesses. Conditions that may be relieved by aromatherapy include painful limbs, muscles and joints due to arthritic or rheumatic disorders, respiratory complaints, digestive disorders, skin conditions, throat and mouth infections, urinary tract infections and problems affecting the hair and scalp. Also, period pains, burns, insect bites and stings, headaches, high blood pressure, feverishness, menopausal symptoms, poor circulation and gout can benefit from aromatherapy. Aromatherapy is of great benefit in relieving stress and stress-related symptoms such as anxiety, insomnia and depression.

Many of the essential oils can be safely used at home and the basic techniques of use can soon be mastered. However, some should only be used by a trained aromatherapist and others must be avoided in certain conditions such as pregnancy. In some circumstances, massage is not considered to be advisable. It is wise to seek medical advice in the event of doubt or if the ailment is more than a minor one.

Consulting a professional aromatherapist

Aromatherapy is a holistic approach to healing hence the practitioner endeavours to build up a complete picture of the patient and his or her lifestyle, nature and family circumstances, as well as noting the symptoms which need to be to be treated. Depending upon the picture that is obtained, the aromatherapist decides upon the essential oil or oils that are most suitable and likely to prove most helpful in the circumstances that prevail. The aromatherapist has a wide ranging knowledge and experience upon which to draw. Many oils can be blended together for an enhanced effect and this is called a 'synergistic blend'. Many aromatherapists offer a massage and/or instruction on the use of the selected oils at home.

Examples of some essential oils

Basil is now grown in many countries of the world although it originates from Africa. The herb has a long history of medicinal and culinary use, and was familiar to the Ancient Egyptian and Greek civilizations. Basil is sacred in the Hindu religion and has many medicinal uses in India and other Eastern countries. The whole plant is subjected to a process of steam distillation to obtain the essential oil used in aromatherapy. Basil has a refreshing, invigorating effect and also has antiseptic properties. It is used in massage, inhalation and baths, and can help to relieve the symptoms of tiredness, colds and respiratory disorders, indigestion and digestive problems, and minor skin wounds and rashes. It can help to alleviate the symptoms of depression although it has a depressive effect if used to excess.

Bergamot oil of bergamot is obtained from a plant that is a native species of some Asian and Eastern countries. The oil was first used and traded in Italy and derives its name from the northern city of Bergamo. In Italian medicine, it was popular as a remedy for feverish illnesses and to expel intestinal worms. It has also been used in cosmetics and perfumes, as the flavouring of Earl Grey tea, and in other foods. The oil is squeezed from the peel of the fruits for use in aromatherapy. It has refreshing, soothing and antiseptic properties, and may be combined with eucalyptus to enhance its effects. It can be used in massage, inhalation and baths, and helps to relieve painful or itchy skin conditions such as psoriasis. It is also used to treat cold sores, mouth and throat infections, shingles, ulcers and symptoms of depression and tiredness.

Eucalyptus is a native species of Australia and Tasmania but is now grown in many countries throughout the world. The plant has a characteristic pungent odour, and the oil obtained from it has disinfectant and antiseptic properties, clears the nasal passages and acts as a painkiller. The leaves and twigs are subjected to a process of steam distillation in order to obtain the essential oil used in aromatherapy. The diluted oil is used for muscular and rheumatic aches and pains, skin disorders such as ringworm, insect bites, headaches and neuralgia, shingles, respiratory and bronchitic infections and fevers. Eucalyptus is used in many household products and in remedies for coughs and colds.

Juniper is a native species of many northern countries and has a long history of medicinal use. It has stimulant, tonic and antiseptic properties with beneficial effects on the skin and the digestive and reproductive organs. It is used to relieve the symptoms of dermatitis, eczema, spots, and dry, sore and chafed skin. Also, it is helpful in the relief of gout and painful rheumatoid arthritis. It is beneficial in the treatment of stress and sleeplessness. In cases of debility, it helps by acting as a tonic for the digestion and boosting the appetite. It can be used in massage, baths and inhalation, and is a useful treatment for cystitis, haemorrhoids (piles) and menstrual problems. Juniper is also used in veterinary medicine and as an ingredient in some toiletries.

Lavender the highly perfumed lavender is a native species of the Mediterranean but has long been popular as a garden plant in Britain and many other countries. It has antiseptic, tonic and relaxing properties, and the essential oil used in aromatherapy is obtained by subjecting the flowers to a process of steam distillation. It is considered to be one of the safest preparations and is used in the treatment of a wide range of disorders. These include minor skin wounds and burns, insect bites, indigestion and digestive problems, muscle pains and strains, cystitis, period pains and premenstrual symptoms, headaches, depression and stress. Lavender is also widely used in perfumes, toiletries and household preparations.

Peppermint is a native plant of Europe with a long history of medicinal use dating back to the ancient civilizations of Egypt, Greece and Rome. Oil of peppermint is obtained by subjecting the flowering parts of the plant to a process of steam distillation. The essential oil of peppermint has a calming effect on the digestive tract and is excellent for the relief of indigestion, colic-type pains, nausea, travel and morning sickness. It is cooling and refreshing, and useful in the treatment of colds, respiratory symptoms and headaches. Peppermint is widely used in remedies for colds and indigestion, as a food flavouring, especially in confectionery, and in toothpaste.

Sage is a native plant of the northern coastal regions of the Mediterranean and has a long history of medicinal and culinary use dating back to the ancient civilizations of Greece and Rome. The essential oil used in aromatherapy is obtained by subjecting the dried leaves to a process of steam distillation. Sage has a stimulating effect upon the circulation and also has tonic, antiseptic, expectorant (when inhaled) and cooling properties. It is used to improve poor circulation, for sore throats, colds and viral infections, bronchitic and catarrhal complaints, rheumatism, arthritic pains, joint sprains and strains, mouth infections and headaches. Sage is widely used as a flavouring in foods and in some household preparations and toiletries.

Ylang ylang is a native species of the Far Eastern islands of Indonesia, the Philippines, Java and Madagascar. To obtain the essential oil used in aromatherapy, the flowers are subjected to a process of steam distillation. The oil has antiseptic and relaxing properties and is also believed to be an aphrodisiac. It has a calming effect on the heartbeat rate and can be used to relieve palpitations, tachycardia, hypertension (raised blood pressure), depression and shock. It has a tonic effect upon the skin and is beneficial in the treatment of nervous complaints. Ylang ylang is used in perfumes and toiletries and as a flavouring in the food industry.

Chiropractic

The word chiropractic originates from two Greek words *kheir*, which means 'hand', and *praktikos*, which means 'practical'. A school of chiropractic was established in about 1895 by a healer called Daniel Palmer (1845–1913). He was able to cure a man's deafness that had occurred when he bent down and felt a bone click. Upon examination Palmer discovered that some bones of the man's spine had become displaced. After successful manipulation the man regained his hearing. Palmer formed the opinion that if there was any displacement in the skeleton this could affect the function of nerves, either increasing or decreasing their action and thereby resulting in a malfunction i.e. a disease.

Chiropractic is used to relieve pain by manipulation and to correct any problems that are present in joints and muscles but especially the spine. Like osteopathy, no use is made of surgery or drugs. If there are any spinal disorders they can cause widespread problems elsewhere in the body such as the hip, leg or arm and can also initiate lumbago, sciatica, a slipped disc or other back problems. It is even possible that spinal problems can result in seemingly unrelated problems such as catarrh, migraine, asthma, constipation, stress, etc. However, the majority of a chiropractor's patients suffer mainly from neck and back pain. People suffering from whiplash injuries sustained in car accidents commonly seek the help of a chiropractor. The whiplash effect is caused when the head is violently wrenched either forwards or backwards at the time of impact.

Another common problem that chiropractors treat is headaches, and it is often the case that tension is the underlying cause as it makes the neck muscles contract. Athletes can also obtain relief from injuries such as tennis elbow, pulled muscles, injured ligaments and sprains, etc. As well as the normal methods of manipulating joints, the chiropractor may decide it is necessary to use applications of ice or heat to relieve the injury.

Children can also benefit from treatment by a chiropractor, as there may be some slight accident that occurs in their early years that can reappear in adult life in the form of back pain. It can easily happen, for example, when a child learns to walk and bumps into furniture, or when a baby falls out of a cot. This could result in some damage to the spine that will show only in adult life when a person experiences back pain. At birth, a baby's neck may be injured or the spine may be strained if the use of forceps is necessary, and this can result in headaches and neck problems as he or she grows to maturity. This early type of injury could also account for what is known as 'growing pains', when the real problem is actually damage that has been done to the bones or muscles. If a parent has any worries it is best to consult a doctor and it is possible that the child will be recommended to see a qualified chiropractor. To avoid any problems in adult life, chiropractors recommend that children have occasional examinations to detect any damage or displacement in bones and muscles.

As well as babies and children, adults of all ages can benefit from chiropractic. There are some people who regularly take painkillers for painful joints or back pain, but this does not deal with the root cause of the pain, only the symptoms that are produced. It is claimed that chiropractic could be of considerable help in giving treatment to these people. Many pregnant women experience backache at some stage during their pregnancy because of the extra weight that is placed on the spine, and they also may find it difficult keeping their balance. At the time of giving birth, changes take place in the pelvis and joints at the bottom of the spine and this can be a cause of back pain. Lifting and carrying babies, if not done correctly, can also damage the spine and thereby make the back painful.

It is essential that any chiropractor is fully qualified and registered with the relevant professional association. At the initial visit, a patient will be for asked details of his or her case history, including the present problem, and during the examination painful and tender areas will be noted and joints will be checked to see whether they are functioning correctly or not. X-rays are frequently used by chiropractors as these help them to make a detailed diagnosis since they can show signs of bone disease, fractures or arthritis as well as the spine's condition. After the initial visit, any treatment will normally begin as soon as the patient has been informed of the chiropractor's diagnosis. If it has been decided that chiropractic therapy will not be of any benefit, the patient will be advised accordingly.

For treatment, underwear and/or a robe will be worn, and the patient will either lie, sit or stand on a specially designed couch. Chiropractors use their hands in a skilful way to effect the different manipulative techniques. If it is decided that manipulation is necessary to treat a painful lumbar joint, the patient will need to lie on his or her side. The upper and lower spine will then be rotated manually but in opposite ways. This manipulation will have the effect of partially locking the joint that is being treated, and the upper leg is usually flexed to aid the procedure. The vertebra that is immediately below or above the joint will then be felt by the chiropractor, and the combination of how the patient is lying, coupled with gentle pressure applied by the chiropractor's hand, will move the joint to its furthest extent of normal movement. There will then be a very quick push applied on the vertebra, which results in its movement being extended further than normal, ensuring that full use of the joint is regained. This is due to the muscles that surround the joint being suddenly stretched, which has the effect of relaxing the muscles of the spine that work upon the joint. This alteration should cause the joint to be able to be used more naturally and should not be a painful procedure.

There can be a variety of effects felt after treatment—some patients may feel sore or stiff, or may ache some time after the treatment, while others will experience the lifting of pain at once. In some cases there may be a need for multiple treatments, perhaps four or more, before improvement is felt. On the whole, problems that have been troubling a patient for a considerable time (chronic) will need more therapy than anything that occurs quickly and is very painful (acute).

Although there is only quite a small number of chiropractors in the UK—yet this numbers is increasing—there is a degree of contact and liaison between them and doctors. It is generally accepted that chiropractic is an effective remedy for bone and muscular problems, and the majority of doctors would be happy to accept a chiropractor's diagnosis and treatment, although the treatment of any general diseases, such as diabetes or asthma, would not be viewed in the same manner.

Herbal Medicine

History of the use of herbal remedies

The medicinal use of herbs is said to be as old as mankind itself. In early civilizations, food and medicine were linked and many plants were eaten for their health-giving properties. In ancient Egypt, the slave workers were given a daily ration of garlic to help fight off the many fevers and infections that were common at that time. The first written records of herbs and their beneficial properties were compiled by the ancient Egyptians. Most of our knowledge and use of herbs can be traced back to the Egyptian priests who also practised herbal medicine. Records dating back to 1500 BC listed medicinal herbs, including caraway and cinnamon.

The ancient Greeks and Romans also carried out herbal medicine, and as they invaded new lands their doctors encountered new herbs and introduced herbs such as rosemary or lavender into new areas. Other cultures with a history of herbal medicine are the Chinese and the Indians. In Britain, the use of herbs developed along with the establishment of monasteries around the country, each of which had its own herb garden for use in treating both the monks and the local people. In some areas, particularly Wales and Scotland, Druids and other Celtic healers are thought to have had an oral tradition of herbalism, where medicine was mixed with religion and ritual.

Over time, these healers and their knowledge led to the writing of the first 'herbals', which rapidly rose in importance and distribution upon the advent of the printing press in the 15th century. John Parkinson of London wrote a herbal around 1630, listing useful plants. Many herbalists set up their own apothecary shops, including the famous Nicholas Culpepper (1616–1654) whose most famous work is *The Complete Herbal and English Physician, Enlarged,* published in 1649. Then in 1812, Henry Potter started a business supplying herbs and dealing in leeches. By this time a huge amount of traditional knowledge and folklore on medicinal herbs was available from Britain, Europe, the Middle East, Asia and the Americas. This promoted Potter to write *Potter's Encyclopaedia of Botanical Drugs and Preparations*, which is still published today.

It was in this period that scientifically inspired conventional medicine rose in popularity, sending herbal medicine into a decline. In rural areas, herbal medicine continued to thrive in local folklore, traditions and practices. In 1864 the National Association (later Institute) of Medical Herbalists was established, to organize training of herbal medicine practitioners and to maintain standards of practice. From 1864 until the early part of this century, the Institute fought attempts to ban herbal medicine and over time public interest in herbal medicine has increased, particularly over the last 20 years. This move away from synthetic drugs is partly due to possible side effects, bad publicity, and, in some instances, a mistrust of the medical and pharmacological industries. The more natural appearance of herbal remedies has led to its growing support and popularity. Herbs from America have been incorporated with common remedies and scientific research into herbs and their active ingredients has confirmed their healing power and enlarged the range of medicinal herbs used today.

Herbal medicine can be viewed as the precursor of modern pharmacology, but today it continues as an effective and more natural method of treating and preventing illness. Globally, herbal medicine is three to four times more commonly practised than conventional medicine.

Forms of herbal preparations

capsule this is a gelatine container for swallowing and holding oils or balsams that would otherwise be difficult to administer due to their unpleasant taste or smell. It is used for cod liver oil and castor oil.
decoction this is prepared using cut, bruised or ground bark and roots placed into a stainless steel or enamel pan (not aluminium) with cold water poured on. The mixture is boiled for 20–30 minutes, cooled and strained. It is best drunk when warm.
herbal dressing this may be a compress or poultice. A compress is

made of cloth or cotton wool soaked in cold or warm herbal decoctions or infusions while a poultice can be made with fresh or dried herbs. Bruised fresh herbs are applied directly to the affected area and dried herbs are made into a paste with water and placed on gauze on the required area. Both dressings are very effective in easing pain, swelling and inflammation of the skin and tissues.

infusion this liquid is made from ground or bruised roots, bark, herbs or seeds, by pouring boiling water onto the herb and leaving it to stand for 10–30 minutes, possibly stirring the mixture occasionally. The resultant liquid is strained and used. Cold infusions may be made if the active principles are yielded from the herb without heat. Today, infusions may be packaged into teabags for convenience.

liquid extract this preparation, if correctly made, is the most concentrated fluid form in which herbal drugs may be obtained and, as such, is very popular and convenient. Each herb is treated by various means dependent upon the individual properties of the herb, e.g. cold percolation, high pressure, evaporation by heat in a vacuum. These extracts are commonly held in a household stock of domestic remedies.

pessary similar to suppositories, but it is used in female complaints to apply a preparation to the walls of the vagina and cervix.

pill probably the best known and most widely used herbal preparation. It is normally composed of concentrated extracts and alkaloids, in combination with active crude drugs. The pill may be coated with sugar or another pleasant-tasting substance that is readily soluble in the stomach.

solid extract this type of preparation is prepared by evaporating the fresh juices or strong infusions of herbal drugs to the consistency of honey. It may also be prepared from an alcoholic tincture base. It is used mainly to produce pills, plasters, ointments and compressed tablets.

suppository this preparation is a small cone of a convenient and easily soluble base with herbal extracts added, which is used to apply medicines to the rectum. It is very effective in the treatment of piles, cancers, etc.

tablet this is made by compressing drugs into a small compass. It is more easily administered and has a quicker action as it dissolves more rapidly in the stomach.

tincture this is the most prescribed form of herbal medicine. It is based on alcohol and, as such, removes certain active principles from herbs that will not dissolve in water, or in the presence of heat. The tincture produced is long-lasting, highly concentrated and only needs to be taken in small doses for beneficial effects. The ground or chopped dried herb is placed in a container with 40 per cent alcohol such as gin or vodka and left for two weeks. The tincture is then decanted into a dark bottle and sealed before use.

Medical terms

In homoeopathy and herbal treatments there are numerous terms used. Listed below are some of the more common terms likely to be encountered in the example herbs provided in this section.

alterative a term given to a substance that speeds up the renewal of the tissues, so that they can carry out their functions more effectively.

anodyne a drug that eases and soothes pain.

anthelmintic a substance that causes the death or expulsion of parasitic worms.

antiperiodic a drug that prevents the return of recurring diseases, e.g. malaria.

antiscorbutic a substance that prevents scurvy and contains necessary vitamins, e.g. vitamin C.

antiseptic a substance that prevents the growth of disease-causing microorganisms, e.g. bacteria, without causing damage to living tissue. It is applied to wounds to cleanse them and prevent infection.

antispasmodic a drug that diminishes muscle spasms.

aperient a medicine that produces a natural movement of the bowel.

aphrodisiac a compound that excites the sexual organs.

aromatic a substance that has an aroma.

astringent a substance that causes cells to contract by losing proteins from their surface. This causes localized contraction of blood vessels and tissues.

balsamic a substance that contains resins and benzoic acid and that is used to alleviate colds and abrasions.

bitter a drug that is bitter-tasting and is used to stimulate the appetite.

cardiac compounds that have some effect on the heart.

carminative a preparation to relieve flatulence and griping.

cathartic a compound that produces an evacuation of the bowels.

cooling a substance that reduces the temperature and cools the skin.

demulcent a substance that soothes and protects the alimentary canal.

deobstruent a compound that is said to clear obstructions, and open the natural passages of the body.

detergent a substance that has a cleansing action, either internally or on the skin.

diaphoretic a term given to drugs that promote perspiration.

diuretics applied to substances that stimulate the kidneys and increase urine and solute production.

emetic a drug that induces vomiting.

emmenagogue a compound that is able to excite the menstrual discharge.

emollient a substance that softens or soothes the skin.

expectorant a group of drugs that are taken to help in the removal of secretions from the lungs, bronchi and trachea.

febrifuge a substance that reduces fever.

galactogogue an agent that stimulates the production of breast milk or increases milk flow.

hydrogogue applied to substances that have the property of removing accumulations of water or serum.

hypnotic drugs or substances that induce sleep.

irritant a general term encompassing any agent that causes irritation of a tissue.

laxative a substance that is taken to evacuate the bowel or soften stools.

mydriatic a compound that cause dilation of the pupil.

nervine a name given to drugs that are used to restore the nerves to their natural state.

narcotic a drug that leads to a stupor and complete loss of awareness.
nutritive compounds that are nourishing to the body.
pectoral applied to drugs that are a remedy in treating chest and lung complaints.
purgative the name given to drugs or other measures that produce evacuation of the bowels. This has normally a more severe effect than aperients or laxatives.
refrigerant a substance that relieves thirst and produces a feeling of coolness.
resolvent a substance that is applied to swellings to reduce them in size.
rubefacient a compound that causes the skin to redden and peel off. Causes blisters and inflammation.
sedative a drug that lessens tension, anxiety and soothes over-excitement of the nervous system.
stimulant a drug or other agent that increases the activity of an organ or system within the body.
stomachic name given to drugs that treat stomach disorders.
styptic applications that check bleeding by blood vessel contraction or by causing rapid blood clotting.
sudorific a drug or agent that produces copious perspiration.
taenicide drugs that are used to expel tapeworms from the body.
tonic substances that are traditionally thought to give strength and vigour to the body and that are said to produce a feeling of wellbeing.
vermifuge a substance that kills, or expels, worms from the intestines.
vulnerary a drug that is said to be good at healing wounds.

Examples of herbs

Aconite *Aconitum napellus. Common name*: Monkshood, blue rocket, friar's cap, wolfsbane.
Occurrence: indigenous to mountain slopes in the Alps and Pyrenees. Introduced into England very early, before 900 AD.
Parts used: the leaves used fresh and the root when dried. It contains

alkaloidal material—aconitine, benzaconine and aconine amongst other compounds.

Medicinal uses: the plant is poisonous and should not be used except under medical advice. It is an anodyne, diaphoretic, febrifuge and sedative. Used for reducing fever and inflammation in the treatment of catarrh, tonsillitis and croup. It may be used in controlling heart spasm.

Administered as: tincture, liniment and occasionally as hypodermic injection.

Anemone wood *Anemone nemorosa. Common name*: Crowfoot, windflower, smell fox.

Occurrence: found in woods and thickets across Great Britain.

Parts used: the root, leaves and juice.

Medicinal uses: this species of plant is much less widely used than it has been previously. It used to be good for leprosy, lethargy, eye inflammation and headaches. An ointment made of the leaves is said to be effective in cleansing malignant ulcers.

Administered as: decoction, fresh leaves and root, ointment.

Anemone pulsatilla *Anemone pulsatilla. Common name*: Pasque flower, meadow anemone, wind flower

Occurrence: found locally in chalk downs and limestone areas of England.

Parts used: the whole herb. It produces oil of anemone upon distillation with water.

Medicinal uses: nervine, antispasmodic, alterative and diaphoretic. It is beneficial in disorders of mucous membranes and of the respiratory and digestive passages. Can be used to treat asthma, whooping cough and bronchitis.

Administered as: fluid extract.

Balm *Melissa officinalis. Common name*: Sweet balm, lemon balm, honey plant, cure-all.

Occurrence: a common garden plant in Great Britain that was naturalized into southern England at a very early period.

Parts used: the herb.
Medicinal uses: as a carminative, diaphoretic, or febrifuge. It can be made into a cooling tea for fever patients and balm is often used in combination with other herbs to treat colds and fever.
Administered as: an infusion.

Belladonna *Atropa belladonna. Common name*: Deadly nightshade, devil's cherries, dwale, black cherry, devil's herb, great morel.
Occurrence: native to central and southern Europe but commonly grows in England.
Parts used: the roots and leaves. The root contains several alkaloid compounds including hyoscyamine, atropine and belladonnine. The same alkaloids are present in the leaves but the amount of each compound varies according to plant type and methods of storing and drying leaves.
Medicinal uses: as a narcotic, diuretic, sedative, mydriatic, antispasmodic. The drug is used as an anodyne in febrile conditions, night sweats and coughs. It is valuable in treating eye diseases and is used as a pain-relieving lotion to treat neuralgia, gout, rheumatism and sciatica. Belladonna is an extremely poisonous plant and should always be used under medical supervision. Cases of accidental poisoning and death are well known. Despite this, it is a valuable drug used to treat a wide range of disease.
Administered as: a liquid extract that is used to produce alcoholic extracts, plasters, liniment, suppositories, tincture and ointment.

Broom *Cytisus scoparius. Common name*: Broom tops, Irish tops, basam, bizzom, browne, brum, bream, green broom.
Occurrence: indigenous to England and commonly found on heathland throughout Great Britain, Europe and northern Asia.
Parts used: the young herbaceous tops that contain sparteine and scoparin as the active components.
Medicinal uses: diuretic and cathartic. The broom tops may be used as a decoction or infusion to aid dropsy, while if the tops are pressed and treated broom juice is obtained. This fluid extract is generally

used in combination with other diuretic compounds. An infusion of broom, agrimony and dandelion root is excellent in remedying bladder, kidney and liver trouble. *Cytisus* should be used carefully as the sparteine has a strong effect on the heart and, depending upon dose, can cause weakness of the heart similar to that caused by hemlock (*Conium maculatum*). Death can occur in extreme cases if the respiratory organ's activity is impaired.

Administered as: fluid extract and infusion.

Chamomile *Anthemis nobilis. Common name*: Roman chamomile, double chamomile, manzanilla (Spanish), maythen (Saxon).
Occurrence: a low-growing plant found wild in the British Isles.
Parts used: the flowers and herb. The active principles therein are a volatile oil, anthemic acid, tannic acid and a glucoside.
Medicinal uses: tonic, stomachic, anodyne and antispasmodic. An infusion of chamomile tea was once thought to be a remedy for hysterical and nervous afflictions in women, as well as an emmenagogue. It has a powerful soothing and sedative effect that is harmless. A tincture is used to cure diarrhoea in children and it is used with purgatives to prevent griping, and as a tonic it helps dropsy. Externally, it can be applied alone or with other herbs as a poultice to relieve pain, swellings, inflammation and neuralgia. Its strong antiseptic properties make it invaluable for reducing swelling of the face due to abscess or injury. As a lotion, the flowers are good for resolving toothache and earache. The herb itself is an ingredient in herb beers. The use of chamomile can be dated back to ancient Egyptian times when they dedicated the plant to the sun because of its extensive healing properties.
Administered as: decoction, infusion, fluid extract and essential oil.

Clover, Red *Trifolium pratense. Common name*: Trefoil, purple clover.
Occurrence: widely distributed in Britain and Europe.
Parts used: the flowers.
Medicinal uses: alterative, sedative, antispasmodic. The fluid extract or infusion are excellent in treating bronchial and whooping coughs.

External application of the herb in a poultice has been used on cancerous growths.

Administered as: fluid extract and infusion.

Coltsfoot *Tussilago farfara*. *Common name*: Coughwort, hallfoot, horsehoof, ass's foot, foals-wort, fieldhove, bullsfoot, donnhove.

Occurrence: commonly found wild on waste ground and riverbanks in Great Britain.

Parts used: the leaves, flowers and root.

Medicinal uses: demulcent, expectorant and tonic. Coltsfoot is one of the most popular cough remedies and is generally taken in conjunction with horehound, marshmallow or ground ivy. It has been called 'Nature's best herb for the lungs' and it was recommended that the leaves be smoked to relieve a cough. Today, it forms the basis of British herb tobacco along with bogbean, eyebright, wood betony, rosemary, thyme, lavender and chamomile, which is said to relieve asthma, catarrh, bronchitis and lung troubles.

Administered as: syrup or smoked when dried.

Comfrey *Symphytum officinale*. *Common name*: Common comfrey, knitbone, knitback, bruisewort, slippery root, gum plant, consolida, ass ear, blackwort.

Occurrence: a native of Europe and temperate Asia but is common throughout England by rivers and ditches.

Parts used: the root and leaves. The roots contain a large quantity of mucilage, choline and allantoin.

Medicinal uses: demulcent, mildly astringent, expectorant and vulnerary. It is frequently used in pulmonary complaints, to soothe intestinal trouble and is a gentle remedy for diarrhoea and dysentery. A strong decoction or tea is administered in cases of internal haemorrhage whether it is the lungs, stomach, bowels or haemorrhoids. Externally, the leaves have been used as a poultice to promote healing of severe cuts, ulcers and abscesses and to reduce swelling, sprains and bruises. Allantoin is known to reduce swelling round damaged or fractured bones, thus allowing healing to occur faster and more thoroughly.

Administered as: a decoction, poultice and liquid extract.

Dandelion *Taraxacum officinale*. *Common name*: Priest's crown, swine's snout.

Occurrence: widely found across the northern temperate zone in pastures, meadows and waste ground.

Parts used: the root and leaves. The main constituents of the root are taraxacin, a bitter substance, and taraxacerin, an acid resin, along with the sugar inulin.

Medicinal uses: diuretic, tonic and slightly aperient. It acts as a general body stimulant, but chiefly acts on the liver and kidneys. Dandelion is used as a bitter tonic in atonic dyspepsia as a mild laxative and to promote increased appetite and digestion. The herb is best used in combination with other herbs and is used in many patent medicines. Roasted dandelion root is also used as a coffee substitute and helps ease dyspepsia, gout and rheumatism.

Administered as: fluid extract, decoction, infusion, tincture, solid extract and juice.

Elder *Sambucus nigra*. *Common name*: black elder, common elder, European elder, pipe tree, bore tree, bour tree.

Occurrence: frequently seen in Europe and Great Britain.

Parts used: the bark, leaves, flowers and berries.

Medicinal uses: the bark is a strong purgative and in large doses is emetic. It has been used successfully in epilepsy, and a tincture of the young bark relieves asthmatic symptoms and croup in children. A tea made from elder roots was highly effective against dropsy. The leaves are used both fresh and dried and contain the alkaloid sambucine, a glucoside called sambunigrin, as well as hydrogenic acid, cane sugar and potassium nitrate amongst other compounds. The leaves are used in preparation of green elder ointment, which is used domestically for bruises, haemorrhoids, sprains, chilblains and applied to wounds. Elder leaves have the same purgative effects as the bark (but produce more nausea) and have expectorant, diaphoretic and diuretic actions.

The elder flowers are either distilled into elderflower water or dried. The water is used in eye and skin lotions as it is mildly astringent and

a gentle stimulant. When infused, the dried flowers make elderflower tea, which is gently laxative, aperient and diaphoretic. It is an old-fashioned remedy for colds and influenza when taken hot, before bed. The tea is also recommended to be drunk before breakfast as a blood purifier. Elder flowers would also be made into a lotion or poultice for use on inflamed areas and into an ointment that was good on wounds, scalds and burns. The ointment was used on the battlefields in World War I and at home for chapped hands and chilblains.
Administered as: an infusion, tincture, ointment, syrup, lotion, distilled water, poultice and dried powder.

Evening primrose *Oenothera biennis*. *Common name*: Tree primrose, sun drop.
Occurrence: native to North America but has been naturalized to British and European gardens.
Parts used: the bark and leaves.
Medicinal uses: astringent, sedative. The drug from this herb is not extensively used but has been of benefit in treating gastro-intestinal disorders, dyspepsia, liver torpor and in female problems in association with pelvic illness. It has also been successfully used in whooping cough and spasmodic asthma.
Administered as: liquid extract.

Fennel *Foeniculum vulgare*. *Common name*: Hinojo, fenkel, sweet fennel, wild fennel.
Occurrence: found wild in most areas of temperate Europe and generally considered indigenous to the shores of the Mediterranean. It is cultivated for medicinal benefit in France, Russia, India and Persia.
Parts used: the seeds, leaves and roots. The roots are rarely used in herbal medicine today. The essential oil is separated by distillation with water. Fennel oil varies in quality and composition dependent upon where, and under what conditions, the fennel was grown.
Medicinal uses: aromatic, stimulant, carminative and stomachic. The herb is principally used with purgatives to allay their tendency to griping, and the seeds form an ingredient of the compound liquorice powder.

Fennel water also acts in a similar manner to dill water in correcting infant flatulence.

Administered as: fluid extract, distilled water, essential oil.

Foxglove *Digitalis purpurea. Common name*: Witch's gloves, dead men's bells, fairy's glove, gloves of Our Lady, bloody fingers, Virgin's glove, fairy caps, folk's glove, fairy thimbles, fair women's plant.

Occurrence: indigenous and widely distributed throughout Great Britain and Europe.

Parts used: the leaves, which contain four important glucosides—digitoxin, digitalin, digitalein and digitonin—of which the first three listed are cardiac stimulants.

Medicinal uses: cardiac tonic, sedative, diuretic. Administering digitalis increases the activity of all forms of muscle tissue, particularly the heart and arterioles. It causes a very high rise in blood pressure and the pulse is slowed and becomes regular. Digitalis causes the heart to contract in size, allowing increased blood flow and nutrient delivery to the organ. It also acts on the kidneys and is a good remedy for dropsy, particularly when it is connected with cardiac problems. The drug has benefits in treating internal haemorrhage, epilepsy, inflammatory diseases and delirium tremens. Digitalis has a cumulative action whereby it is liable to accumulate in the body and then have poisonous effects. It should only be used under medical advice. Digitalis is an excellent antidote in aconite poisoning when given as a hypodermic injection.

Administered as: tincture, infusion, powdered leaves, injection.

Golden rod *Solidago virgaurea. Common name*: Verge d'or, solidago, woundwort, Aaron's Rod.

Occurrence: this is a plant normally found wild in woods in Great Britain, Europe, Central Asia and North America but it is also a common garden plant.

Parts used: the leaves contain tannin, with some bitter and astringent chemicals that are unknown.

Medicinal uses: aromatic, stimulant, carminative. This herb is astrin-

gent and diuretic and is highly effective in curing gravel and urinary stones. It aids weak digestion, stops sickness and is very good against diphtheria. As a warm infusion it is a good diaphoretic drug and is used as such to help painful menstruation and amenorrhoea (absence or stopping of menstrual periods).
Administered as: fluid extract, infusion, spray.

Hemlock *Conium maculatum*. *Common name*: Herb bennet, spotted conebane, musquash root, beaver poison, poison hemlock, poison parsley, spotted hemlock, vex, vecksies.
Occurrence: common in hedges, meadows, waste ground and stream banks throughout Europe and also found in temperate Asia and north Africa.
Parts used: the leaves, fruits and seeds. The most important constituent of hemlock leaves is the alkaloid coniine, which is poisonous, with a disagreeable odour. Other alkaloids in the plant include methylconiine, conhydrine, pseudoconhydrine, ethyl piperidine.
Medicinal uses: sedative, antispasmodic, anodyne. The drug acts on the centres of motion and causes paralysis and so it is used to remedy nervous motor excitability, e.g. teething, cramp and muscle spasms of the larynx and gullet.

When inhaled, hemlock is said to be good in relieving coughs, bronchitis, whooping cough and asthma. The method of action of *Conium* means it is directly antagonistic to the effects of strychnine, from nux vomica (*Strychnos nux-vomica*), and it is used as an antidote to strychnine poisoning and similar poisons. Hemlock has to be administered with care as narcotic poisoning may result from internal application and overdoses induce paralysis, with loss of speech and depression of respiratory function leading to death. Antidotes to hemlock poisoning are tannic acid, stimulants, e.g. coffee, mustard and castor oil.
Administered as: powdered leaves, fluid extract, tincture, expressed juice of the leaves and solid extract.

Honeysuckle *Lonicera caprifolium*. *Common name*: Dutch honeysuckle, goat's leaf, perfoliate honeysuckle.

Occurrence: it grows freely in Europe, Great Britain and through the northern temperate zone.

Parts used: the dried flowers and leaves.

Medicinal uses: expectorant, laxative. A syrup made of the flowers is used for respiratory diseases and asthma. A decoction of the leaves is laxative and is also good against diseases of the liver and spleen, and in gargles.

Administered as: syrup, decoction.

Juniper *Juniperus communis*.

Occurrence: a common shrub native to Great Britain and widely distributed through many parts of the world.

Parts used: the berry and leaves.

Medicinal uses: the oil of juniper obtained from the ripe berries is stomachic, diuretic and carminative and is used to treat indigestion and flatulence as well as kidney and bladder diseases. The main use of juniper is in dropsy, and aiding other diuretic herbs to ease the disease.

Administered as: essential oil from berries, essential oil from wood, fluid extract, liquid extract, solid extract.

Larch *Pinus larix*. *Common name*: *Larix europaea*, *Abies larix*, *Larix decidua*, *Laricus cortex*, European larch, Venice turpentine.

Occurrence: indigenous to hilly regions of central Europe, but was introduced into Great Britain in 1639.

Parts used: the inner bark, which contains tannic acid, larixinic acid and turpentine.

Medicinal uses: stimulant, diuretic, astringent, balsamic and expectorant. It is very useful as an external application for eczema and psoriasis. However, it is mainly used as a stimulant expectorant in chronic bronchitisand for internal haemorrhage and cystitis. Larch turpentine has also been suggested as an antidote in cyanide or opium poisoning and has been used as a hospital disinfectant.

Administered as: fluid extract or syrup.

Liquorice *Glycyrrhiza glabra. Common name*: Licorice, lycorys, *Liquiriha officinalis.*
Occurrence: a shrub native to southeast Europe and southwest Asia and cultivated in the British Isles.
Parts used: the root. The chief compound in the root is glychrrhizin along with sugar, starch, gum, tannin and resin.
Medicinal uses: demulcent, pectoral, emollient. A very popular and well-known remedy for coughs, consumption and chest complaints. Liquorice extract is included in cough lozenges and pastilles, with sedatives and expectorants. An infusion of bruised root and flax (linseed) is good for irritable coughs, sore throats and laryngitis. Liquorice is used to a greater extent as a medicine in China and other eastern countries. The herb is used by brewers to give colour to porter and stout and is employed in the manufacture of chewing or smoking tobacco.
Administered as: powdered root, fluid extract, infusion, solid extract.

Meadowsweet *Spiraea ulmaria. Common name*: Meadsweet, dolloff, queen of the meadow, bridewort, lady of the meadow.
Occurrence: a common wild plant in the British Isles, found growing in meadows or woods.
Parts used: the herb.
Medicinal uses: aromatic, astringent, diuretic, alterative. This herb is good against diarrhoea, stomach complaints and blood disorders. It is highly recommended for children's diarrhoea and dropsy and was used as a decoction in wine to reduce fevers. Meadowsweet makes a pleasant everyday drink when infused and sweetened with honey. It is also included in many herb beers.
Administered as: infusion, decoction.

Nettle *Urtica dioica, Urtica urens. Common name*: Common nettle, stinging nettle.
Occurrence: widely distributed throughout temperate Europe and Asia, Japan, South Africa and Australia.
Parts used: the whole herb, which contains formic acid, mucilage, mineral salts, ammonia and carbonic acid.

Medicinal uses: astringent, stimulating, diuretic, tonic. The herb is anti-asthmatic and the juice of the nettle will relieve bronchial and asthmatic troubles, as will the dried leaves when burnt and inhaled. The seeds are taken as an infusion or in wine to ease consumption or ague. Nettles are used widely as a food source and are made into puddings, tea, beer, juice and used as a vegetable. A hair tonic or lotion can also be made from the herb. In the Highlands of Scotland, they were chopped, added to egg white and applied to the temples as a cure for insomnia.

Administered as: expressed juice, infusion, decoction, seeds, dried herb, dietary item.

Peppermint *Mentha piperita. Common name: Brandy mint, curled mint, balm mint.*

Occurrence: found across Europe, was introduced into Britain and grows widely in damp places and waste ground.

Parts used: the herb and distilled oil. The plant contains peppermint oil, which is composed of menthol, menthyl acetate and isovalerate, menthone, cineol, pinene and limonene. The medicinal qualities are found in the alcoholic chemicals.

Medicinal uses: stimulant, antispasmodic, carminative, stomachic, oil of peppermint is extensively used in both medicine and commerce. It is good in dyspepsia, flatulence, colic and abdominal cramps. The oil allays sickness and nausea, is used for chorea and diarrhoea but is normally used with other medicines to disguise unpalatable tastes and effects. Peppermint water is in most general use and is used to raise body temperature and induce perspiration. Peppermint tea can help ward off colds and influenza at an early stage, can calm heart palpitations and is used to reduce the appetite.

Administered as: infusion, distilled water, spirit, essential oil, fluid extract.

Primrose *Primula vulgaris.*

Occurrence: a common wild flower found in woods, hedgerows and pastures throughout Great Britain.

Parts used: the root and whole herb. Both parts of the plant contain a

fragrant oil called primulin and the active principle saponin.
Medicinal uses: astringent, antispasmodic, vermifuge, emetic. It was
formerly considered to be an important remedy in muscular rheumatism, paralysis and gout. A tincture of the whole plant has sedative
effects and is used successfully in extreme sensitivity, restlessness and
insomnia. Nervous headaches can be eased by treatment with an infusion of the root, while the powdered dry root serves as an emetic.
An infusion of Primrose flowers is excellent in nervous headaches
and an ointment can be made out of the leaves to heal and salve
wounds and cuts.
Administered as: infusion, tincture, powdered root and ointment.

Ragwort *Senecio jacobaea. Common name*: St James's wort, stinking
nanny, staggerwort, ragweed, dog standard, cankerwort,
stammerwort, fireweed.
Occurrence: an abundant wild plant, widely distributed over Great
Britain, Europe, Siberia and northwest India.
Parts used: the herb.
Medicinal uses: diaphoretic, detergent, emollient, cooling, astringent.
The leaves were used as emollient poultices, while the expressed juice
of the herb was utilized as a wash in burns, eye inflammation, sores
and cancerous ulcers. It has been successful in relieving rheumatism,
sciatica, gout and in reducing inflammation and swelling of joints
when applied as a poultice. Ragwort makes a good gargle for ulcerated throats and mouths and a decoction of its root is said to help
internal bruising and wounds. The herb was previously thought to be
able to prevent infection. This plant is poisonous to cattle and should
be removed from their pastures. The alkaloids in the ragwort have
cumulative effects in the cattle and low doses of the chemical eaten
over a period of time can built up to a critical level, where the cattle
show obvious symptoms and then die. It is uncertain if sheep are also
susceptible to this chemical.
Administered as: poultice, infusion and decoction.
Rosemary *Rosmarinus officinalis. Common name*: Polar plant, com-
pass-weed, compass plant, romero, *Rosmarinus coronarium*.

Occurrence: native to the dry hills of the Mediterranean, from Spain westward to Turkey. A common garden plant in Britain, having been cultivated prior to the Norman Conquest.

Parts used: the herb and root. Oil of rosemary is distilled from the plant tops and used medicinally. Rosemary contains tannic acid, a bitter principle, resin and a volatile oil.

Medicinal uses: tonic, astringent, diaphoretic, stimulant. The essential oil is also stomachic, nervine and carminative and cures many types of headache. It is mainly applied externally as a hair lotion that is said to prevent baldness and the formation of dandruff. The oil is used externally as a rubefacient and is added to liniments for fragrance and stimulant properties. Rosemary tea can remove headache, colic, colds and nervous diseases and may also lift nervous depression.

Administered as: infusion, essential oil and lotion.

Sorrel *Rumex acetosa*. *Common name*: Garden sorrel, green sauce, sour grabs, sour suds, cuckoo sorrow, cuckoo's meate, gowke-meat.

Occurrence: indigenous to Britain and found in moist meadows throughout Europe.

Parts used: the leaves, dried and fresh.

Medicinal uses: refrigerant, diuretic, antiscorbutic. Sorrel is given as a cooling drink in all febrile conditions and can help correct scrofulous deposits. Its astringent qualities meant it was formerly used to stop haemorrhages and was applied as a poultice on cutaneous tumours. Sorrel juice and vinegar are said to cure ringworm, while a decoction was made to cure jaundice, ulcerated bowel, and gravel and stone in the kidneys.

Administered as: expressed juice, decoction, poultice and dried leaves.

Tansy *Tanacetum vulgare*. *Common name*: Buttons.

Occurrence: a hardy perennial plant, commonly seen on waste ground all over Europe and Great Britain.

Parts used: the herb. It contains the chemicals tanacetin, tannic acid, a volatile oil, thujone, sugar and a colouring matter among others.

Medicinal uses: anthelmintic, tonic, emmenagogue, stimulant. Tansy is largely used for expelling worms from children. The herb is also used for slight fevers, for allaying spasms and as a nervine drug. In large doses, the herb is violently irritant and induces venous congestion of the abdominal organs. In Scotland, an infusion was administered to cure gout. Tansy essential oil, when given in small doses, has helped in epilepsy and has also been used externally to help some eruptive diseases of the skin. Bruised fresh leaves can reduce swelling and relieve sprains, as can a hot infusion used as a poultice.

Administered as: essential oil, infusion, poultice, fresh leaves, solid extract.

Thyme *Thymus vulgaris*. *Common name*: Garden or common thyme, tomillo.

Occurrence: cultivated in temperate countries in northern Europe.

Parts used: the herb. Thyme gives rise to oil of thyme after distillation of the fresh leaves. This oil contains the phenols, thymol and carvacrol, as well as cymene, pinene and borneol.

Medicinal uses: antiseptic, antispasmodic, tonic, carminative. The fresh herb, in syrup, forms a safe cure for whooping cough, as is an infusion of the dried herb. The infusion or tea is beneficial for catarrh, sore throat, wind spasms, colic and in allaying fevers and colds. Thyme is generally used in conjunction with other remedies in herbal medicine.

Administered as: fluid extract, essential oil and infusion.

Valerian *Valeriana officinalis*. *Common name*: all-heal, great wild valerian, amantilla, setwall, sete-wale, capon's tail.

Occurrence: found throughout Europe and northern Asia. It is common in England in marshy thickets, riverbanks and ditches.

Parts used: the root, which contains a volatile oil, two alkaloids called chatarine and Valerianine as well as several unidentified compounds.

Medicinal uses: powerful nervine, stimulant, carminative anodyne and antispasmodic herb. It may be given in all cases of nervous debility and irritation as it is not narcotic. The expressed juice of the fresh root has been used as a narcotic in insomnia and as an anticonvulsant in epilepsy. The oil of valerian is of use against cholera and in strengthening the eyesight. A herbal compound containing valerian was given to civilians during the Second World War, to reduce the effects of stress caused by repeated air raids and to minimize damage to health.

Administered as: fluid extract, tincture, essential oil, expressed juice.

Witch hazel *Hamamelis virginiana. Common name*: Spotted alder, winterbloom, snapping hazelnut.

Occurrence: native to the United States of America and Canada. *Parts used*: the dried bark, both fresh and dried leaves. The leaves contain tannic and gallic acids, volatile oil and an unknown bitter principle. The bark contains tannin, gallic acid, a physterol, resin, fat and other bitter and odorous bodies.

Medicinal uses: astringent, tonic, sedative. Valuable in stopping internal and external haemorrhages and in treating piles. Mainly used for bruises, swelling, inflammation and tumours as a poultice. It may also be utilized for diarrhoea, dysentery and mucous discharges. A decoction is used against tuberculosis, gonorrhoea, menorrhagia and the debilitated state resulting from abortion. Tea made from the bark or leaves aids bleeding of the stomach, bowel complaints and may be given as an injection for bleeding piles. Witch hazel is used to treat varicose veins as a moist poultice, as an extract to ease burns, scalds and insect and mosquito bites, and to help inflammation of the eyelids.

Administered as: liquid extract, injection, tincture, lotion, ointment, suppositories, poultice, infusion and decoction.

Homeopathy

Introduction

The aim of homeopathy is to cure an illness or disorder by treating the whole person rather than merely concentrating on a set of symptoms. Hence, in homeopathy the approach is holistic, and the overall state of health of the patient, especially his or her emotional and psychological wellbeing, is regarded as being very significant. A homeopath notes the symptoms that the person wishes to have cured, but also takes time to discover other signs or indications of disorder that the patient may regard as being less important. The reasoning behind this is that illness is a sign of disorder or imbalance within the body. It is believed that the whole 'make-up' of a person determines, to a great extent, the type of disorders to which that individual is prone and the symptoms likely to occur. A homeopathic remedy must be suitable both for the symptoms and the characteristics and temperament of the patient. Hence, two patients with the same illness may be offered different remedies according to their individual natures. One remedy may also be used to treat different groups of symptoms or ailments.

Homoeopathic remedies are based on the concept that 'like cures like', an ancient philosophy that can be traced back to the 5th century BC when it was formulated by Hippocrates. In the early 1800s, this idea awakened the interest of a German doctor, Samuel Hahnemann, who believed that the medical practices at that time were too harsh and tended to hinder rather than aid healing. Hahnemann observed that a treatment for malaria, based on an extract of cinchona bark (quinine), actually produced symptoms of this disease when taken in a small dose by a healthy person. Further extensive studies convinced him that the production of symptoms was the body's way of combating illness. Hence, to give a minute dose of a substance that stimulated the symptoms of an illness in a healthy person, could be used to fight that illness in someone who was sick. Hahnemann conducted numerous trials (called 'provings') giving minute doses of substances to healthy people and recording the symptoms produced. Eventually, these very dilute remedies were given to people with illnesses, often with very encouraging results.

Modern homeopathy is based upon the work of Hahnemann, and the medicines derived from plant, mineral and animal sources are used in extremely dilute amounts. Indeed it is believed that the curative properties are enhanced by each dilution because impurities that might cause unwanted side effects are lost. Substances used in homeopathy are first soaked in alcohol to extract their essential ingredients. This initial solution, called the 'mother tincture' is diluted successively either by factors of ten (called the 'decimal scale' and designated X), or 100 (the 'centesimal scale' and designated C). Each dilution is shaken vigorously before further ones are made and this is thought to make the properties more powerful by adding energy at each stage, while impurities are removed. The thorough shakings of each dilution are said to energize or 'potentiate' the medicine. The remedies are made into tablets or may be used in the form of ointment, solutions, powders, suppositories, etc. High potency (i.e. more dilute) remedies are used for severe symptoms and lower potency (less dilute) for milder ones.

The homeopathic view is that during the process of healing, symptoms are redirected from more important to less important body systems. It is also held that healing is from innermost to outermost parts of the body and that more recent symptoms disappear first, this being known as the 'law of direction of cure'. Occasionally, symptoms may worsen initially when a homeopathic remedy is taken, but this is usually short-lived and is known as a 'healing crisis.' It is taken to indicate a change and that improvement is likely to follow. Usually, with a homeopathic remedy, an improvement is noticed fairly quickly although this depends upon the nature of the ailment, health, age and wellbeing of the patient and potency of the remedy.

A first homeopathic consultation is likely to last about 1 hour so that the specialist can obtain a full picture of the patient's medical history and personal circumstances. On the basis of this information, the homeopathic doctor decides on an appropriate remedy and potency (which is usually 6C). Subsequent consultations are generally shorter and full advice is given on how to store and take the medicine. It is widely accepted that homeopathic remedies are very safe and non-addictive but they are covered by the legal requirements governing all medicines and should be obtained from a recognized source.

Potency table for homeopathic medicines

The centesimal scale
1C = 1/100	$(1/100^1)$	of mother tincture
2C = 1/10 000	$(1/100^2)$	of mother tincture
3C = 1/1 000 000	$(1/100^3)$	of mother tincture
6C = 1/1 000 000 000 000	$(1/100^6)$	of mother tincture

The decimal scale
1X = 1/10	$(1/10^1)$	of mother tincture
2X = 1/100	$(1/10^2)$	of mother tincture
6X = 1/1 000 000	$(1/10^6)$	of mother tincture

The development of homeopathy

The Greek physician, Hippocrates, who lived several hundred years before the birth of Christ (460–370 BC), is regarded as the founding father of all medicine. The Hippocratic Oath taken by newly qualified doctors in orthodox medicine binds them to an ethical code of medical practice in honour of Hippocrates. Hippocrates believed that disease resulted from natural elements in the world in which people lived. This contrasted with the view that held sway for centuries that disease was some form of punishment from the gods or God. He believed that it was essential to observe and take account of the course and progress of a disease in each individual, and that any cure should encourage that person's own innate healing power. Hippocrates embraced the idea of 'like being able to cure like' and had many remedies that were based on this principle. Hence in his practice and study of medicine he laid the foundations of the homeopathic approach although this was not to be appreciated and developed for many centuries.

During the period of Roman civilization a greater knowledge and insight into the nature of the human body was developed. Many herbs and plants were used for healing by people throughout the world, and much knowledge was gained and handed down from generation to generation. However, the belief persisted that diseases were caused by supernatural or divine forces. It was not until the early 1500s that a Swiss doctor, Paracelsus (1493–1541) put forward the view that disease resulted from external environmental forces. He also believed that plants and natural substances held the key to healing and embraced the 'like can cure like' principle. One of his ideas, known as the Doctrine of Signatures, was that the appearance of a plant, or the substances it contained, gave an idea of the disorders it could cure.

In the succeeding centuries, increased knowledge was gained about the healing properties of plants and the way the human body worked. In spite of this, the methods of medical practice were extremely harsh and there is no doubt that many people suffered needlessly and died due to the treatment they received. It was against this background that Samuel Hahnemann, (1755–1843) the founding father of modern homeopathy, began his work as a doctor in the late 1700s. In his early writings, Hahnemann criticized the severe practices of medicine and advocated a healthy diet, clean living conditions and high standards of hygiene as a means of improving health and warding off disease. In 1790, he became interested in quinine, extracted from the bark of the cinchona tree, which was known to be an effective treatment for malaria. He tested the substance first on himself, and later on friends and close family members and recorded the results, and these early experiments were called 'provings'. The results led him to conduct many further investigations and provings of other natural substances, during the course of which he rediscovered and established the principle of like being able to cure like.

By 1812, the principle and practice of homeopathy, based on the work of Hahnemann, had become established and many other doctors adopted the homeopathic approach. Hahnemann himself become a teacher in homeopathy at the University of Leipzig and published many important writings—the results of his years of research. He continued to practice, teach and conduct research throughout his life, especially in producing more dilute remedies that were succussed or shaken at each stage and were found to be more potent. Although his work was not without its detractors, Hahnemann had attracted a considerable following by the 1830s. In 1831, there was a widespread cholera epidemic in central Europe for which Hahnemann recommended treatment with camphor. Many people were cured, including Dr Frederick Quin, (1799–1878), a medical practitioner at that time. He went on to establish the first homeopathic hospital in London in 1849. A later resurgence of cholera in Britain enabled the effectiveness of camphor to be established beyond doubt, as the numbers of people cured at the homeopathic hospital were far greater than those treated at other hospitals.

In the United States of America, homeopathy became firmly established in the early part of the 19th century and there were several eminent practitioners who further enhanced knowledge and practice. These included Dr Constantine Hering (1800–1880), who formulated the Laws of Cure, explaining how symptoms affect organ systems and move from one part of the body to another as a cure occurs. Dr James Tyler Kent (1849–1916) introduced the idea of constitutional types, which is now the basis of classical homeopathy, and advocated the use of high potency remedies.

In the later years of the 19th century, a fundamental split occurred in the practice of homeopathy, which was brought about by Dr Richard Hughes (1836–1902), who worked in London and Brighton. He insisted that physical symptoms and the nature of the disease itself were the important factors rather than the holistic approach, based on the make-up of the whole individual person. Hughes rejected the concept of constitutional types and advocated the use of low-potency remedies. Although he worked as a homeopath, his approach was to attempt to make homeopathy more scientific and to bring it closer to the practices of conventional medicine. Some other homeopathic doctors followed the approach of Hughes, and the split led to a collapse in faith in the whole practice of homeopathy during the early part of the century. However, as the century advanced, homeopathy regained its following and respect. Conventional medicine and homeopathy have continued to advance, and there is now a greater sympathy and understanding between the practitioners in both these important disciplines.

Among homeopathic remedies there are a small number of fundamental, regularly used compounds that are effective in treating many complaints. These are described below.

Basic remedies

Argenticum nitricum

Argent nit; silver nitrate, devil's stone, lunar caustic, hellstone.

Silver nitrate is obtained from the mineral acanthite, which is a natural ore of silver. White silver nitrate crystals are derived from a chemical solution of the mineral ore, and these are used to make the homeopathic remedy. Silver nitrate is poisonous in large doses and has antiseptic and caustic properties. In the past it was used to clean out wounds and prevent infection. In homeopathy, it is used to treat states of great anxiety, panic, fear or apprehension about a forthcoming event, e.g. taking an examination, having to perform a public role (speech-making, chairing a public meeting, acting, singing), going for an interview or any activity involving scrutiny and criticism by others. It was also used as a remedy for digestive complaints including indigestion, abdominal pain, wind, nausea and also for headache. Often, there is a longing for sweet 'comfort' or other types of food. Argent nit. may be given for laryngitis, sore throat and hoarseness, eye inflammation such as conjunctivitis and for period pains. Other types of pain, asthma and warts may benefit from argent nit.

Often, a person experiences symptoms mainly on the left side and these are worse for heat and at night. Also, they are made worse by anxiety and overwork, emotional tension and resting on the left side. Pains are made worse with talking and movement. Symptoms improve in cold or cool fresh air and are relieved by belching. Pains are helped by applying pressure to the painful part. People suitable for argent nit. are quick-witted and rapid in thought and action. They may appear outgoing and happy but are a prey to worry, anxiety and ungrounded fears that make them tense. All the emotions are quick to surface and argent nit. people are able to put on an impressive performance. They enjoy a wide variety of foods, particularly salty and sweet things, although these may upset the digestion. They have a fear of heights, crowds, of being burgled, of failure, and arriving late for an appointment. They also have a fear of serious illness, dying and madness.

Argent nit. people are generally slim and full of restless energy and tension. They may have deeply etched features and lines on the skin that make them appear older than their actual age.

Arsenicum album
Arsen alb; white arsenic trioxide.
This is a widely used homeopathic remedy, the source being white arsenic trioxide derived from arsenopyrite, a metallic mineral ore of arsenic. Arsenic has been known for centuries as a poison and was once used as a treatment for syphilis. White arsenic trioxide used to be given to improve muscles and skin in animals such as horses. It is used to treat acute conditions of the digestive system and chest and mental symptoms of anxiety and fear. Hence it is a remedy for diarrhoea and vomiting caused by eating the wrong kinds of food, or food poisoning or over-indulgence in alcohol. Also, for dehydration in children following gastroenteritis or feverish illness. It is a remedy for asthma and breathing difficulty, mouth ulcers, carbuncle (a collection of boils), dry, cracked lips, burning skin, inflamed, watering stinging eyes and psoriasis. Also, for sciatica, shingles, sore throat and painful swallowing, candidiasis (fungal infection) of the mouth and motion sickness. There may be oedema (retention of fluid) showing as a puffiness around the ankles.

An ill person who benefits from arsen alb. experiences burning pains but also feels cold. The skin may be either hot or cold to the touch. The symptoms are worse for cold in any form, including cold food and drink, and between midnight and 3 a.m. They are worse on the right side and if the person is near the coast. Symptoms improve with warmth (including warm drinks), gentle movement and lying down with the head raised. People suitable for arsen alb. are precise, meticulous and ambitious and loathe any form of disorder. They are always immaculately dressed and everything in their life is neat and tidy. However, they tend to have great worries, especially about their financial security and their own health and that of their family. They fear illness and dying, loss of financial and personal status, being burgled, darkness and the supernatural. Arsen alb. people have strongly held views and do not readily tolerate contrary opinions or those with a more relaxed or disordered lifestyle. They enjoy a variety of different foods, coffee and alcoholic drinks. They are usually thin, with delicate, fine features and pale skin that may show worry lines. Their movements tend to be rapid and their manner serious and somewhat restless, although they are always polite.

Calcarea carbonica

Calc. carb; calcium carbonate.

This important homeopathic remedy is made from powdered mother-of-pearl, the beautiful, translucent inner layer of oyster shells. Calcium is an essential mineral in the body, being especially important for the healthy development of bones and teeth. The calc. carb. remedy is used to treat a number of different disorders especially those relating to bones and teeth, but also certain skin conditions and symptoms relating to the female reproductive system. It is a remedy for weak or slow growth of bones and teeth and fractures that take a long time to heal. Also, for teething problems in children, pains in bones, teeth and joints, headaches and eye inflammations affecting the right side, and ear infections with an unpleasant-smelling discharge. Premenstrual syndrome, heavy periods and menopausal disorders are helped by calc. carb, and also chapped skin and eczema.

Calc. carb. may be used as a remedy for verruca (a type of wart) and thrush infections. People who benefit from calc. carb. are very sensitive to the cold, particularly in the hands and feet and tend to

sweat profusely. They suffer from fatigue and anxiety, and body secretions (sweat and urine) smell unpleasant. Children who benefit from
calc. carb. have recurrent ear, nose and throat infections, especially
tonsillitis and glue ear. Symptoms are made worse by draughts and
cold, damp weather and also at night. They are worse when the person first wakens in the morning and for physical exercise and sweating. In women, symptoms are worse premenstrually. They improve in
warm, dry weather and are better later on in the morning and after
the person has eaten breakfast. People suitable for calc. carb. are often overweight or even obese with a pale complexion. They are shy
and very sensitive, quiet in company and always worried about what
other people think of them. Calc. carb. people are hard-working, conscientious and reliable and easily upset by the suffering of others.
They need constant reassurance from friends and family and tend to
feel that they are a failure. Usually, calc. carb. people enjoy good health
but have a tendency for skeletal weakness. They enjoy a wide variety
of different foods and tend to overeat, but are upset by coffee and
milk. They are afraid of dying and serious illness, the supernatural,
madness, being a failure and becoming poor and they tend to be claustrophobic.

Graphites
Graphite; black pencil lead
Graphite is a form of carbon that is the basis of all life. It is found in
older igneous or metamorphic rocks, such as granite and marble and
is mined for its industrial uses, e.g. in batteries, motors, pencil leads,
cleaning and lubricating fluids. It was investigated and proved by
Hahnemann after he learned that it was being used by some factory
workers to heal cold sores. The powder used in homeopathy is ground
graphite and it is mainly used for skin disorders that may be caused
by metabolic imbalances and stomach ulcers. It is a remedy for eczema, psoriasis, acne, rough, dry skin conditions with pustules or blisters, scarring and thickened cracked nails and cold sores. Also, for
stomach ulcers due to a thinning or weakness in the lining of the
stomach wall, problems caused by excessive catarrh, loss of hair and

cramping pains or numbing of the feet and hands. In women it is used to treat some menstrual problems. The symptoms are worse in draughty, cold and damp conditions and for eating sweet meals or sea foods. Also, the use of steroids for skin complaints and, in women, during menstruation. Symptoms are often worse on the left side. They improve with warmth, as long as the air is fresh and it is not stuffy, when it is dark and with eating and sleep. People suitable for graphites are usually well built and may be overweight, often having dark hair. They like to eat well but lack physical fitness and sweat or flush with slight exertion. They are prone to dry, flaky skin conditions that may affect the scalp. Graphites people are usually lethargic and may be irritable, lacking in concentration for intellectual activities. They are prone to mood swings and subject to bouts of weeping, especially when listening to music. A graphites person feels that he or she is unlucky and is inclined to self-pity, often feeling fearful and timid.

Ignatia amara
Agnate; strychnos Ignatii, St Ignatius' bean
Ignatia amara is a large tree that is native to the Philippine Islands, China and the East Indies. The tree has many branches and twining stems and produces stalked white flowers. Later, seed pods are produced, each containing ten to twenty large, oval seeds, that are about one inch long and are embedded in pulp. The seeds are highly poisonous and contain strychnine, which affects the central nervous system. Similar active constituents and properties are found in *Nux vomica*. The tree is named after the founder of the Jesuits, Ignatius Loyola (1491–1556), and Spanish priests belonging to this order brought the seeds to Europe during the 1600s. The homeopathic remedy is made from the powdered seeds and is used especially for emotional symptoms. It is used for grief, bereavement, shock and loss, particularly when a person is having difficulty coming to terms with his or her feelings and is inclined to suppress the natural responses. Accompanying symptoms include sleeplessness, anger and hysteria. Similar emotional and psychological problems are helped by this remedy, including anxiety and fear especially of appearing too forward to others, a

tendency to burst into fits of crying, self-doubt, pity, blame and depression. Nervous tension headaches and digestive upsets, feverish symptoms, chills and pains in the abdomen may be helped by *Ignatia*. Some problems associated with menstruation, especially sharp pains or absence of periods, are relieved by this remedy as are conditions with changeable symptoms. These are worse in cold weather or conditions, with emotional trauma, being touched, for smoking and drinking coffee. They improve with warmth, moving about, eating, lying on the side or area that is painful and after passing urine.

The person for whom *Ignatia* is suitable is usually female and with a tendency towards harsh, self-criticism and blame; she is usually a creative, artistic person, highly sensitive but with a tendency to suppress the emotions. She is perceptive and intelligent but inclined to be hysterical and subject to erratic mood swings. Typically, the person expects a high standard in those she loves. The person enjoys dairy products, bread and sour foods but sweets, alcoholic drinks and fruit upset her system. She is afraid of crowds, tends to be claustrophobic, and fears being burgled. Also, she is afraid of being hurt emotionally, and is very sensitive to pain. The person is usually dark-haired and of slim build with a worried expression and prone to sighing, yawning and excessive blinking.

Lachesis
Trigonocephalus lachesis; lachesis muta, venom of the bushmaster or Surukuku snake
This South African snake produces a deadly venom that may prove instantly fatal due to its effects upon the heart. The venom causes the blood to thin and flow more freely, hence increasing the likelihood of haemorrhage. Even a slight bite bleeds copiously with a risk of blood poisoning or septicaemia. The snake is a ferocious hunter and its African name, Surukuku describes the sound it makes while in pursuit of prey. The properties of the venom were investigated in the 1800s by the eminent American homeopathic doctor, Constantine Hering , who tested and proved the remedy on himself. It is effective in treating a variety of disorders, particularly those relating to the blood cir-

culation and where there is a risk of blood poisoning or septicaemia. It is used to treat varicose veins and problems of the circulation indicated by a bluish tinge to the skin. The remedy is useful for those suffering from a weak heart or angina, palpitations and an irregular, fast or weak pulse. There may be symptoms of chest pain and breathing difficulty. It is of great benefit in treating uterine problems, particularly premenstrual congestion and pain that is relieved once the period starts. Also, this is an excellent remedy for menopausal symptoms, especially hot flushes, and for infections of the bladder and rectum. It is used to treat conditions and infections where symptoms are mainly on the left side, such as headache or stroke when the left side is involved. Also, as a treatment for sore throats and throat infections, tonsillitis, lung abscess, boils, ulcers, wounds that only heal slowly, vomiting due to appendicitis and digestive disorders, fevers with chills and shivering, nosebleeds and bleeding piles.

It is used to treat severe symptoms of measles and serious infections including scarlet fever and smallpox. Symptoms are made worse for touch and after sleep and by tight clothing. They are worse for hot drinks and baths, and exposure to hot sun or direct heat in any form. For women, symptoms are worse during the menopause. They improve with being out in the fresh air and drinking cold drinks and with release of normal bodily discharges. People suitable for *Lachesis* tend to be intelligent, creative, intense and ambitious. They have strong views about politics and world affairs and may be impatient of the views of others. They may be somewhat self-centred, possessive and jealous, which can cause problems in close relationships with others. They dislike being tied down and so may be reluctant to commit themselves to a relationship. *Lachesis* people have a liking for sour pickled foods, bread, rice and oysters and alcoholic drinks. They like coffee, but hot drinks and wheat-based food tends to upset them. They have a fear of water, people they do not know, being burgled and of dying or being suffocated. *Lachesis* people may be somewhat overweight and are sometimes red-haired and freckled. Alternatively, they may be thin and dark-haired, pale and with a lot of energy. Children tend to be somewhat jealous of others and

possessive of their friends, which can lead to naughty or trying behaviour.

Lycopodium clavatum

Lycopodium; club moss, wolf's claw, vegetable sulphur, stagshorn
moss, running pine
This plant is found throughout the northern hemisphere, in high moor-
lands, forests and mountains. The plant produces spore cases on the
end of upright forked stalks, which contain the spores. These produce yellow dust or powder that is resistant to water and was once
used as a coating on pills and tablets to keep them separate from one
another. The powder was also used as a constituent of fireworks. It
has been used medicinally for many centuries, as a remedy for digestive disorders and kidney stones in Arabian countries and in the treatment of gout. The powder and spores are collected by shaking the
fresh, flowering stalks of the plant and its main use in homeopathy is
for digestive and kidney disorders. It is used to treat indigestion, heartburn, the effects of eating a large meal late at night, sickness, nausea,
wind, bloatedness and constipation. Also, in men, for kidney stones,
with the production of a red-coloured urine containing a sand-like
sediment and enlarged prostate gland. It is used in the treatment of
some problems of male impotence and bleeding haemorrhoids or piles.
Symptoms that occur on the right side are helped by *Lycopodium*,
and the patient additionally tends to crave sweet, comfort foods.
Nettlerash, psoriasis affecting the hands, fatigue due to illness and
ME (Myalgic encephalomyelitis), some types of headache, cough and
sore throat are relieved by this remedy. It is used to relieve emotional
states of anxiety, fear and apprehension caused by chronic insecurity,
or relating to forthcoming events such as taking an examination or
appearing in public (stage fright). Also, night terrors, sleeplessness,
shouting or talking in the sleep and being frightened on first waking
up can all benefit from this treatment.

The symptoms are worse between 4 p.m. and 8 p.m. and in warm,
stuffy rooms and with wearing clothes that are too tight. They are
also worse in the early morning between 4 a.m. and 8 a.m., for eating

too much and during the Spring. They improve outside in cool fresh air, after a hot meal or drink and with loosening tight clothing, with light exercise and at night. People suitable for *Lycopodium* tend to be serious, hard-working and intelligent, often in professional positions. They seem to be self-possessed and confident but are, in reality, rather insecure with a low self-opinion. They are impatient of what they perceive as being weakness and are not tolerant or sympathetic of illness. *Lycopodium* people are sociable but may keep their distance and not get involved; they may be sexually promiscuous. They have a great liking for sweet foods of all kinds and enjoy hot meals and drinks. They are easily filled but may carry on eating regardless of this and usually complain of symptoms on the right side. *Lycopodium* people are afraid of being left on their own, of failure in life, of crowds, darkness and the supernatural and tend to be claustrophobic. They are often tall, thin and pale with receding hair or hair that turns grey early in life. They may be bald, with a forehead lined with worry lines and a serious appearance. They tend to have weak muscles and are easily tired after physical exercise. They may have a tendency to unconsciously twitch the muscles of the face and to flare the nostrils.

Mercurius solubilis
Merc sol; quicksilver
The mineral cinnabar, which is found in volcanic crystalline rocks, is an important ore of mercury and is extracted for a variety of uses, including dental fillings and in thermometers. Mercury is toxic in large doses, and an affected person produces copious quantities of saliva and suffers repeated bouts of vomiting. Mercury has been used since ancient times and was once given as a remedy for syphilis. A powder of precipitate of mercury is obtained from dissolving liquid mercury in a dilute solution of nitric acid, and this is the source of the remedy used in homeopathy. It is used as a remedy for conditions that produce copious bodily secretions that often smell unpleasant, with accompanying symptoms of heat or burning and a great sensitivity to temperature. It is used as a remedy for fevers with profuse, unpleasant sweating, bad breath, inflammation of the gums, mouth ulcers,

candidiasis (thrush) of the mouth, infected painful teeth and gums and excessive production of saliva. Also, for a sore infected throat, tonsillitis, mumps, discharging infected ear and a congested severe headache and pains in the joints. It is good for eye complaints including severe conjunctivitis, allergic conditions with a running nose, skin complaints that produce pus-filled pustules, spots and ulcers, including varicose ulcers. The symptoms are made worse by extremes of heat and cold and also for wet and rapidly changing weather. They are worse at night and for sweating and being too hot in bed.

Symptoms improve for rest and in comfortable temperatures where the person is neither too hot nor too cold. People suitable for merc. sol. tend to be very insecure although they have an outwardly calm appearance. They are cautious and reserved with other people and consider what they are about to say before speaking so that conversation may seem laboured. Merc. sol. types do not like criticism of any kind and may suddenly become angry if someone disagrees with their point of view. They tend to be introverted but their innermost thoughts may be in turmoil. They tend to be hungry and enjoy bread and butter, milk and other cold drinks but dislike alcohol with the exception of beer. They usually do not eat meat and do not have a sweet tooth. They dislike coffee and salt. Merc. sol. people often have fair hair with fine, unlined skin and an air of detachment. They are afraid of dying and of mental illness leading to insanity, and worry about the wellbeing of their family. They fear being burgled and are afraid or fearful during a thunderstorm.

Natrum muriaticum

Natrum mur; common salt, sodium chloride

Salt has long been prized for its seasoning and preservative qualities, and Roman soldiers were once paid in salt, such was its value. (Salary comes from the latin word *salarium*, which refers to this practice). Sodium and chlorine are essential chemicals in the body, being needed for many metabolic processes, particularly the functioning of nerve tissue. In fact, there is seldom a need to add salt to food as usually enough is present naturally in a healthy, well-balanced diet. (An exception is when people are working very hard physically in a hot climate and losing a lot of salt in sweat). However, people and many other mammals frequently have a great liking for salt. If the salt/water balance in the body is disturbed, a person soon becomes very ill and may even die.

In ancient times, salt was usually obtained by boiling sea water, but natural evaporation around the shallow edges of salt lakes results in deposits of rock salt being formed. Rock salt is the usual source of table salt and also of the remedy used in homeopathy. This remedy has an effect on the functioning of the kidneys and the salt/water balance of body fluids, and is used to treat both mental and physical symptoms. Emotional symptoms that benefit from natrum mur. include sensitivity and irritability, tearfulness and depression, suppressed grief and premenstrual tension. Physical ailments that respond to this remedy are often those in which there is a thin, watery discharge of mucus and in which symptoms are made worse by heat. Hence natrum mur. is used in the treatment of colds with a runny nose or other catarrhal problems. Also, for some menstrual and vaginal problems, headaches and migraines, cold sores, candidiasis (thrush) of the mouth, mouth ulcers, inflamed and infected gums and bad breath. Some skin disorders are helped by natrum mur. including verruca (a wart on the foot), warts, spots and boils and cracked, dry lips. It may be used in the treatment of fluid retention with puffiness around the face, eyelids and abdomen, etc, urine retention, constipation, anal fissure, indigestion, anaemia and thyroid disorders (goitre).

When ill, people who benefit from this remedy feel cold and shivery but their symptoms are made worse, or even brought on, by heat. Heat, whether from hot sun and fire or a warm, stuffy room exacerbate the symptoms, which also are made worse in cold and thundery weather. They are worse on the coast from the sea breeze, and in the morning between 9 and 11 o'clock. Too much physical activity and the sympathy of others exacerbate the symptoms. They improve in the fresh, open air and for cold applications or a cold bath or swim. Also, sleeping on a hard bed and sweating and fasting make the symptoms better.

People suitable for natrum mur. are often women who are highly sensitive, serious-minded, intelligent and reliable. They have high ideals and feel things very deeply, being easily hurt and stung by slights and criticism. They need the company of other people but, being so sensitive, can actually shun them for fear of being hurt. They are afraid of mental illness leading to loss of self-control and insanity and of dying. Also, they fear the dark, failure in work, crowds, being burgled and have a tendency to be claustrophobic. They worry about being late and are fearful during a thunderstorm. Natrum. mur. people tend to become introverted and react badly to the criticism of others. They are highly sensitive to the influence of music, which easily moves them to tears. Natrum mur. people are usually of squat or solid build with dark or fairish hair. They are prone to reddened, watery eyes as though they have been crying, and a cracked lower lip. The face may appear puffy and shiny with an air of stoicism.

Nux vomica

Strychnos nux vomica; poison nut, Quaker buttons

The strychnos nux vomica tree is a native of India but also grows in Burma, Thailand, China and Australia. It produces small, greenish-white flowers and later, apple-sized fruits, containing small, flat, circular pale seeds covered in fine hair. The seeds, bark and leaves are highly poisonous, containing strychnine, and have been used in medicine for many centuries. In medieval times, the seeds were used as a treatment for the plague. Strychnine has severe effects upon the nervous system but in minute amounts can help increase urination and aid digestion. The seeds are cleaned and dried and used to produce the homeopathic remedy. Nux vomica is used in the treatment of a variety of digestive complaints including cramping, colicky abdominal pains, indigestion, nausea and vomiting, diarrhoea and constipation. Also, indigestion or stomach upset caused by over-indulgence in alcohol or rich food and piles that cause painful contractions of the rectum. Sometimes, these complaints are brought on by a tendency to keep emotions, particularly anger, suppressed and not allowing it to show or be expressed outwardly. Nux vomica is a remedy for irritability, headache and migraine, colds, coughs and influenza-like symptoms of fever, aching bones and muscles and chills and shivering. It is a useful remedy for women who experience heavy, painful periods that may cause fainting, morning sickness during pregnancy and pain in labour. It is also used to treat urinary frequency and cystitis.

The type of person who benefits from this remedy is frequently under stress and experiences a periodic flare-up of symptoms. The person may be prone to indigestion and heartburn, gastritis and stomach ulcer and piles or haemorrhoids. The person usually has a tendency to keep everything bottled up but has a passionate nature and is liable to outbursts of anger. Nux vomica people are very ambitious and competitive, demanding a high standard of themselves and others and intolerant of anything less than perfection. They enjoy challenges and using their wits to keep one step ahead. Often, they are to be found as managers, company directors, scientists, etc, at the cutting edge of their particular occupation. They are ungracious and irritable when ill and cannot abide the criticism of others. This type of person is afraid of being a failure at work and fears or dislikes crowded public places. He or she is afraid of dying. The person enjoys rich, fattening foods containing cholesterol and spicy meals, alcohol and coffee although these upset the digestive system. Symptoms are worse in cold, windy, dry weather and in winter and between 3 and 4 a.m. They are aggravated by certain noises, music, bright lights and touch, eating (especially spicy meals) and with overwork of mental faculties. Nux vomica people usually look serious, tense and are thin with a worried expression. They have sallow skin and tend to have dark shadows beneath the eyes.

Phosphorus
Phos; white phosphorus
Phosphorus is an essential mineral in the body, found in the genetical material (DNA), bones and teeth. White phosphorus is extremely flammable and poisonous and was once used in the manufacture of matches and fireworks. Due to the fact that it tends to catch fire

spontaneously when exposed to air, it is stored under water. In the past it has been used to treat a number of disorders and infectious diseases such as measles. In homeopathy, the remedy is used to treat nervous tension caused by stress and worry, with symptoms of sleeplessness, exhaustion and digestive upset. Often there are pains of a burning nature in the chest or abdomen. It is a remedy for vomiting and nausea, heartburn, acid indigestion, stomach ulcer and gastroenteritis. It is also used to treat bleeding, e.g. from minor wounds, the gums, nosebleeds, gastric and profuse menstrual bleeding.

Severe coughs that may be accompanied by retching, vomiting and production of a blood-tinged phlegm are treated with phos. as well as some other severe respiratory complaints. These include pneumonia, bronchitis, asthma and laryngitis. Styes that tend to recur and poor circulation may also be helped by phos. Symptoms are worse in the evening and morning and before or during a thunderstorm. They are also made worse for too much physical activity, hot food and drink and lying on the left side. Symptoms improve in the fresh open air and with lying on the back or right side. They are better after sleep or when the person is touched or stroked. People who need phos. do not like to be alone when ill and improve for the sympathy and attention of others. They are warm, kind, affectionate people who are highly creative, imaginative and artistic. They enjoy the company of other people and need stimulation to give impetus to their ideas. Phos. people have an optimistic outlook, are full of enthusiasm but sometimes promise much and deliver little. They are very tactile and like to be touched or stroked and offered sympathy when unhappy or unwell. They enjoy a variety of different foods but tend to suffer from digestive upsets. Phos. people are usually tall, slim and may be dark or fair-haired, with an attractive, open appearance. They like to wear brightly coloured clothes, and are usually popular, having many friends. They have a fear of illness, especially cancer, and of dying and also of the dark and supernatural forces. They are apprehensive of water and fear being a failure in their work. Thunderstorms make them nervous.

Pulsatilla nigricans

Pulsatilla; *Anemone pratensis*, meadow anemone

This attractive plant closely resembles *Anemone pulsatilla*, the pasque flower, which is used in herbal medicine, but has smaller flowers. *Anemone pratensis* is a native of Germany, Denmark and Scandinavia and has been used medicinally for hundreds of years. The plant produces beautiful deep purple flowers with orange centres and both leaves and flowers are covered with fine, silky hairs. The whole fresh plant is gathered and made into a pulp and liquid is extracted to make the remedy used in homeopathy. It is used to treat a wide variety of disorders with both physical and mental symptoms. It is a useful remedy for ailments in which there is a greenish-yellowish discharge. Hence it is used for colds and coughs and sinusitis with the production of profuse catarrh or phlegm. Also, eye infections with discharge such as styes and conjunctivitis. Digestive disorders are helped by pulsatilla, particularly indigestion, heartburn, nausea and sickness caused by eating too much fatty or rich food. The remedy is helpful for female disorders in which there are a variety of physical and emotional symptoms. These include premenstrual tension, menstrual problems, menopausal symptoms and cystitis, with accompanying symptoms of mood swings, depression and tearfulness. It is a remedy for headaches and migraine, swollen glands, inflammation and pain in the bones and joints as in rheumatic and arthritic disorders, nosebleeds, varicose veins, mumps, measles, toothache, acne, frequent urination and incontinence.

Symptoms are worse at night or when it is hot, and after eating heavy, rich food. Symptoms improve out in the cool fresh air and with gentle exercise such as walking. The person feels better after crying and being treated sympathetically by others. Pulsatilla people are usually women who have a mild, passive nature and are kind, gentle and loving. They are easily moved to tears by the plight of others and love animals and people alike. The person yields easily to the requests and demands of others and is a peacemaker who likes to avoid a scene. An outburst of anger is very much out of character and a pulsatilla person usually has many friends. The person likes rich and sweet foods, although these may upset the digestion, and dislikes spicy meals. Pulsatilla people may fear darkness, being left alone, dying and any illness leading to insanity. They are fearful of crowds, the supernatural and tend to be claustrophobic. Usually, they are fair and blue-eyed with clear, delicate skin that blushes readily. They are attractive and slightly overweight or plump.

Sepia officinalis
Sepia; ink of the cuttlefish
Cuttlefish ink has been used since ancient times, both for medicinal purposes and as a colour in artists' paint. The cuttlefish has the ability to change colour to blend in with its surroundings and squirts out the dark brown/black ink when threatened by predators. Sepia was known to Roman physicians who used it as a cure for baldness. In homeopathy it is mainly used as an excellent remedy for women experiencing menstrual and menopausal problems. It was investigated and proved by Hahnemann in 1834. It is used to treat premenstrual tension, menstrual pain and heavy bleeding, infrequent or suppressed periods, menopausal symptoms such as hot flushes and postnatal depression. Physical and emotional symptoms caused by an imbalance of hormones are helped by sepia. Also, conditions in which there is extreme fatigue or exhaustion with muscular aches and pains. Digestive complaints, including nausea and sickness, abdominal pain and wind, caused by eating dairy products, and headaches with giddiness and nausea are relieved by sepia. Also, it is a remedy for incontinence, hot, sweaty feet and verruca (a wart on the foot). A woman often experiences pelvic, dragging pains frequently associated with prolapse of the womb. Disorders of the circulation, especially varicose veins and cold extremities benefit from sepia.

Symptoms are worse in cold weather and before a thunderstorm and in the late afternoon, evening and early in the morning. Also, before a period in women and if the person receives sympathy from others. The symptoms are better with heat and warmth, quick vigorous movements, having plenty to do and out in the fresh open air.

People suitable for sepia are usually, but not exclusively, women. They tend to be tall, thin and with a yellowish complexion and are rather self-contained and indifferent to others. Sepia people may become easily cross, especially with family and close friends, and may harbour resentment. In company, they make a great effort to appear outgoing and love to dance. A woman may be either an externally hard, successful career person or someone who constantly feels unable to cope, especially with looking after the home and family. Sepia people have strongly held beliefs and cannot stand others taking a contrary opinion. When ill, they hate to be fussed over or have the sympathy of others. They like both sour and sweet foods and alcoholic drinks but are upset by milk products and fatty meals. They harbour deep insecurity and fear being left alone, illness resulting in madness and loss of their material possessions and wealth. One physical attribute is that they often have a brown mark in the shape of a saddle across the bridge of the nose.

Silicea terra
Silicea; silica.
Silica is one of the main rock-forming minerals and is also found in living things where its main function is to confer strength and resilience. In homeopathy, it is used to treat disorders of the skin, nails and bones and recurring inflammations and infections, especially those that occur because the person is somewhat run-down or has an inadequate diet. Also, some disorders of the nervous system are relieved by silicea. The homeopathic remedy used to be derived from ground flint or quartz but is now prepared by chemical reaction. The remedy is used for catarrhal infections such as colds, influenza, sinusitis, ear infections including glue ear. Also, for inflammations producing pus such as a boil, carbuncle, abscess, stye, whitlow (infection of the finger nail) and peritonsillar abscess. It is beneficial in helping the natural expulsion of a foreign body such as a splinter in the skin. It is a remedy for a headache beginning at the back of the head and radiating forwards over the right eye and for stress-related conditions of over-work and sleeplessness.

Symptoms are worse for cold, wet weather, especially when clothing is inadequate, draughts, swimming and bathing, becoming chilled after removing clothes and in the morning. They are better for warmth and heat, summer weather, warm clothing, particularly a hat or head covering and not lying on the left side. People who are suitable for silicea tend to be thin with a fine build and pale skin. They often have thin, straight hair. They are prone to dry, cracked skin and nails and may suffer from skin infections. Silicea people are usually unassuming, and lacking in confidence and physical stamina. They are conscientious and hard-working to the point of working too hard once a task has been undertaken. However, they may hesitate to commit themselves through lack of confidence and fear of responsibility. Silicea people are tidy and obsessive about small details. They may feel 'put upon', but lack the courage to speak out, and may take this out on others who are not responsible for the situation. They fear failure and dislike exercise due to physical weakness, often feeling mentally and physically exhausted. They enjoy cold foods and drinks.

Sulphur
Sulphur; flowers of sulphur, brimstone.
Sulphur has a long history of use in medicine going back to very ancient times. Sulphur gives off sulphur dioxide when burnt, which smells unpleasant ('rotten eggs' odour) but acts as a disinfectant. This was used in medieval times to limit the spread of infectious diseases. Sulphur is deposited around the edges of hot springs and geysers and where there is volcanic activity. Flowers of sulphur, which is a bright yellow powder, is obtained from the natural mineral deposit and is used to make the homeopathic remedy. Sulphur is found naturally in all body tissues and, in both orthodox medicine and homeopathy, is used to treat skin disorders. It is a useful remedy for dermatitis, eczema, psoriasis and a dry, flaky, itchy skin or scalp. Some digestive disorders benefit from sulphur especially a tendency for food to rise back up to the mouth and indigestion caused by drinking milk. Sulphur is helpful in the treatment of haemorrhoids or piles, premenstrual and menopausal symptoms, eye inflammations such as

conjunctivitis, pain in the lower part of the back, catarrhal colds and coughs, migraine headaches and feverish symptoms.

Some mental symptoms are helped by this remedy particularly those brought about by stress or worry including depression, irritability, insomnia and lethargy. When ill, people who benefit from sulphur feel thirsty rather than hungry and are upset by unpleasant smells. The person soon becomes exhausted and usually sleeps poorly at night and is tired through the day. The symptoms are worse in cold, damp conditions, in the middle of the morning around 11 a.m. and in stuffy, hot, airless rooms. Also, for becoming too hot at night in bed and for wearing too many layers of clothes. Long periods of standing and sitting aggravate the symptoms and they are worse if the person drinks alcohol or has a wash. Symptoms improve in dry, clear, warm weather and for taking exercise. They are better if the person lies on the right side.

Sulphur people tend to look rather untidy and have dry, flaky skin and coarse, rough hair. They may be thin, round-shouldered and in-clined to slouch or be overweight, round and red-faced. Sulphur peo-ple have lively, intelligent minds full of schemes and inventions, but are often useless on a practical level. They may be somewhat self-centred with a need to be praised, and fussy over small unimportant details. They enjoy intellectual discussion on subjects that they find interesting and may become quite heated although the anger soon subsides. Sulphur people are often warm and generous with their time and money. They enjoy a wide range of foods but are upset by milk and eggs. They have a fear of being a failure in their work, of heights and the supernatural.

Additional homeopathic medicines in common use

Aconitum nepalese (aconite, monkshood, wolfsbane, friar's cap, mousebane)
Actea racemosa (black snakeroot, rattleroot, bugbane, rattleweed, squaw root)
Allium (Spanish onion)

Apis mellifica (the honey bee)

Arnica montana (arnica; leopard's bane, sneezewort)

Atropa belladonna (belladonna; deadly nightshade, black cherry, devil's cherries, naughty man's cherries, devil's herb)

Aurum metallicum (aurum met; gold)

Bryonia alba (bryonia; European white bryony, black-berried white bryony, wild hops)

Calcarea fluorica (calc. fluor; fluorite, calcium fluoride, fluoride of lime)

Calcarea phosphorica (calc. phos; phosphate of lime, calcium phosphate)

Calendula officinalis (calendula; marigold, garden marigold)

Cantharis vesicatoria (cantharis; Spanish fly)

Carbo vegetablis (carbo veg; vegetable charcoal)

Chamomilla (chamomile; common chamomile, double chamomile)

China officinalis (cinchona succiruba; china, Peruvian bark, Jesuit's bark)

Citrullus colocynthus (colocynthis; bitter cucumber, bitter apple)

Cuprum metallicum (cuprum met; copper)

Daphne mezereum (daphne; spurge laurel, wild pepper, spurge olive, flowering spurge, dwarf bay)

Drosera rotundifolia (drosera; sundew, youthwort, red rot, moor grass)

Euphrasia officinalis (euphrasia; eyebright)

Ferrum phosphoricum (ferrum phos; phosphate of iron, iron phosphate)

Gelsemium sempervirens (gelsemium; yellow jasmine, false jasmine, Carolina jasmine, wild woodbine)

Guaiacum offinale (guaiac; resin of lignum vitae)

Hamamelis virginiana hamamelis (witch hazel; spotted alder, snapping hazelnut, winterbloom)

Hepar sulphuris calcareum (hepar sulph; sulphide of calcium)

Hypericum perforatum (hypericum, St John's wort)

Ipecacuanha (ipecac; cephalis ipecacuanha, psychotria ipeca-cuanha, the ipecac plant)

Kalium bichromicum (kali bich; potassium dichromate, potassium bichromate)

Kalium iodatum (kali iod; kali hydriodicum, potassium iodide)

Kalium phosphoricum (kali phos; potassium phosphate, phosphate of potash)

Ledum palustre (ledum; marsh tea, wild rosemary)

Rhus toxicodendron (rhus tox; rhus radicaris, American poison ivy, poison oak, poison vine)

Ruta graveolens (ruta grav; rue, garden rue, herbygrass, ave-grace, herb-of-grace, bitter herb)

Tarentula cubensis (tarentula cub; Cuban tarentula)

Thuja occidentalis (thuja; tree of life, yellow cedar, arbor vitae, false white cedar)

Urtica urens (urtica; stinging nettle)

Glossary of terms used in homeopathy

aggravations a term first used by Dr Samuel Hahnemann to describe an initial worsening of symptoms experienced by some patients, on first taking a homeopathic remedy, before the condition improved. In modern homeopathy this is known as a'healing crisis'. To prevent the occurrence of aggravations, Hahnemann experimented with further dilutions of remedies and, in particular, vigorous shaking (succussing) of preparations at each stage of the process.

allopathy a term first used by Dr Samuel Hahnemann meaning 'against disease'. It describes the approach of conventional medicine, which is to treat symptoms with a substance or drug with an opposite effect in order to suppress or eliminate them. This is called the Law of Contraries and is in direct contrast to the 'like can cure like,' the Law of Similars or *Similia Similibus Curentur* principle, which is central to the practice of homeopathy.

centesimal scale of dilution the scale of dilution used in homeopathy based on one part (or drop) of the remedy in 99 parts of the diluent liquid (a mixture of alcohol and water).

classical the practice of homeopathy based on the work of Dr Samuel Hahnemann and further developed and expanded by other practitioners, particularly Dr Constantine Hering and Dr James Tyler Kent.

constitutional prescribing and constitutional types the homeopathic concept, based on the work of Dr James Tyler Kent, that prescribing should be based on the complete make-up of a person, including physical and emotional characteristics, as well as on the symptoms of a disorder.

decimal scale of dilution the scale of dilution used in homeopathy based on one part (or drop) of the remedy in nine parts of the diluent liquid (a mixture of alcohol and water).

healing crisis the situation in which a group of symptoms first become worse after a person has taken a homeopathic remedy, before they improve and disappear. The occurrence of a healing crisis is taken to indicate a change and that improvement is likely to follow. It is usually short-lived, (*see also* aggravations).

homeopathy the system of healing based on the principle of 'like can cure like' and given its name by Samuel Hahnemann. The word is derived from the Greek *homeo* for similar and *pathos* for suffering, or 'like disease'.

laws of cure, law of direction of cure three concepts or 'laws' formulated by Dr Constantine Hering to explain the means by which symptoms of disease are eliminated from the body in homeopathy.
1.Symptoms move in a downwards direction.
2.Symptoms move from the inside of the body outwards.
3.Symptoms move from more important vital organs and tissues tothose of less importance.

Hering was also responsible for the view in homeopathy that more recent symptoms disappear first before ones that have been present for a longer time. Hence symptoms are eliminated in the reverse order of their appearance.

materia medica detailed information about homeopathic remedies, listed alphabetically and includes details of the symptoms that may respond to each remedy, based on previous research and experience. Details about the source of each remedy are also included. This information is used by a homeopathic doctor when deciding upon the best remedy for each particular patient and group of symptoms.

miasm a chronic constitutional weakness that is the aftereffect of an underlying suppressed disease that has been present in a previous generation or earlier in the life of an individual. The concept of miasm was formulated by Samuel Hahnemann who noted that some people were never truly healthy but always acquired new symptoms of illness. He believed that this was due to a constitutional weakness that he called a miasm, which may have been inherited and was caused by an illness in a previous generation. These theories were put forward in his research writings entitled *Chronic Diseases*. Three main miasms were identified, psora, sycosis and syphilis.

modalities a term applied to the responses of the patient, when he or she feels better or worse, depending upon factors in the internal and external environment. These are unique from one person to another depending upon the individual characteristics that apply at the time, although there are common features within each constitutional type. Modalities include responses, fears and preferences to temperature, weather, foods, emotional responses and relationships, etc, which all contribute to a person's total sense of wellbeing. Modalities are particularly important when a person has symptoms of an illness in prescribing the most beneficial remedy.

mother tincture (symbol O) the first solution obtained from dissolving a substance in a mixture of alcohol and water (usually in the ratio of $^9/_{10}$ pure alcohol to $^1/_{10}$ distilled water). The mother tincture is subjected to further dilutions and succussions (shakings) to produce the homeopathic remedies.

nosode a term used to describe a remedy prepared from samples of infected diseased tissue, often to treat or prevent a particular illness. They were first investigated by Wilhelm Lux, not without considerable controversy. Examples are *Medorrhinum and Tuberculinum.*

organon *The Organon of Rationale Medicine.* One of the most important works of Samuel Hahnemann, published in Leipzig in 1810, in which he set out the principles and philosophy of modern homeopathy. The *Organon* is considered to be a classic work and basic to the study of homeopathy.

polycrest a remedy suitable for a number of illnesses, disorders or symptoms.

potency the dilution or strength of a homeopathic remedy. Dr Samuel Hahnemann discovered that by further diluting and succussing (shaking) a remedy, it became more effective or potent in bringing about a cure. It is held that the process of diluting and shaking a remedy releases its innate energy or dynamism, even though none of the original molecules of the substance may remain. Hence the greater the dilution of a remedy, the stronger or more potent it becomes. Hahnemann called his new dilute solutions 'potentizations'.

potentiate the release or transfer of energy into a homeopathic solution by succussing or vigorous shaking of the mixture.

principle of vital force 'vital force' was the term given by Samuel Hahnemann to the inbuilt power or ability of the human body to maintain health and fitness and to fight off illness. Illness is believed to be the result of stresses that cause an imbalance in the vital force, and assail all people throughout life and include inherited, environmental and emotional factors. The symptom of this 'disorder' is illness, and this is held to be the physical indication of the struggle of the body's vital force to regain its balance. A person with a strong vital force will tend to remain in good health and to fight off illness. A person with a weak vital force is more likely to suffer from long-term, recurrent symptoms and illnesses. Homoeopathic remedies are believed to act upon the vital force, stimulating it to heal the body and restore the natural balance.

provings the term given by Samuel Hahnemann to experimental trials he carried out to test the reactions of healthy people to homeopathic substances. These trials were carried out under strictly controlled conditions (in advance of the modern scientific approach), and the symptoms produced were meticulously recorded. Quinine was the substance that Hahnemann first investigated in this way, testing it initially on himself and then on close friends and family members. He continued over the next few years to investigate and prove many other substances, building up a wealth of information on each one about the reactions and symptoms it produced. After conducting this research, Hahnemann went on carefully to prescribe the remedies to those who were sick. Provings are still carried out in modern homeopathy to test new substances that may be of value as remedies. Usually, neither the prescribing physician nor those taking the substance—the 'provers'—know the identity of the material or whether they are taking a placebo.

psora one of three miasms identified by Samuel Hahnemann believed to be caused by suppression of scabies. Psora was believed to have an inherited element or to be caused by suppression of an earlier infection in a particular individual.

Schussler tissue salts Wilhelm Heinrich Schussler was a German homeopathic doctor who introduced the Biochemic Tissue Salt system in the late 1800s. Schussler believed that many symptoms and ailments resulted from the lack of a minute, but essential, quantity of a mineral or tissue salt. He identified twelve such tissue salts that he regarded as essential and believed that a cure could be obtained from replacing the deficient substance. Schussler's work was largely concentrated at the cell and tissue level rather than embracing the holistic view of homeopathy.

similia similibus curentur the founding principle of homeopathy that 'like can cure like' or 'let like be treated by like', which was first put forward by Hippocrates, a physician of ancient Greece. This principle excited the interest of Paracelsus in the Middle Ages, and was later restated and put into practice by Samuel Hahnemann with the development of homeopathy.

simillimum a homeopathic remedy that in its natural state is able to produce the same symptoms as those being exhibited by the patient.

succussion vigorous shaking of a homeopathic remedy at each stage of dilution, along with banging the container and holding it against a hard surface, therebycausing further release of energy.

sycosis one of the three major miasms identified by Samuel

Hahnemann and believed to result from a suppressed gonorrhoeal infection. Sycosis was believed to have an inherited element or to be due to suppression of an earlier infection in a particular individual.

syphilis the third of the three major miasms identified by Samuel Hahnemann believed to result from a suppressed syphilis infection. Syphilis was believed to have an inherited element or to be due to suppression of an earlier infection in a particular individual.

trituration the process, devised by Samuel Hahnemann, of rendering naturally insoluble substances soluble so that they can be made available as homeopathic remedies. The process involves repeated grinding down of the substance with lactose powder until it becomes soluble. The substance usually becomes soluble at the third process of trituration. Each trituration is taken to be the equivalent of one dilution in the centesimal scale. Once the substance has been rendered soluble, dilution can proceed in the normal way.

Massage

As long ago as 3000 BC massage was used as a therapy in the Far East, making it one of the most ancient treatments used by the human race. In 5 BC in ancient Greece, Hippocrates recommended that to maintain health a massage using oils should be taken daily after a perfumed bath. The physicians there were well used to treating people who suffered from pain and stiffness in the joints.

Massage increased in popularity when, in the 19th century, Per Henrik Ling, a Swedish athlete, created the basis for what is now known as Swedish massage. Swedish massage is a combination of relaxing effects and exercises that work on the joints and muscles, but it is still based on the form that was practised in ancient times. More recently, a work was published by George Downing in the 1970s called *The Massage Book,* and this introduced a new concept in the overall technique of massage, that the whole person's state should be assessed by the therapist and not solely the physical side. The emotional and mental states should be part of the overall picture. Also combined in his form of massage were the methods used in reflexology and shiatsu, and this was known as therapeutic massage. The aim of this is to use relaxation, stimulation and invigoration to promote good health.

This massage is commonly used to induce general relaxation, so that any tension or strain experienced in the rush of daily life can be eased and eliminated. It is found to be very effective, working on the mind as well as the body. It can be used to treat people with hypertension (high blood pressure), sinusitis, headaches, insomnia and hyperactivity, including people who suffer from heart ailments or circulatory disorders. At the physical level, massage is intended to help the body make use of food and to eliminate the waste materials, as well as stimulating the nervous and muscular system and the circulation of blood. Neck and back pain are conditions from which many people suffer, particularly if they have not been sitting correctly, such as in a slightly stooped position with their shoulders rounded. People whose day-to-day work involves a great deal of physical activity, such as dancers and athletes, can also derive a great deal of benefit from the use of massage. Stiffness can be a problem that they have after training or working, and this is relieved by encouraging the toxins that gather in the muscles to disperse. Massage promotes a feeling of calmness and serenity, and this is particularly beneficial to people who frequently suffer from bouts of depression or anxiety. Once the worry and depression have been dispelled, people are able to deal with their problems much more effectively and, being able to do so, will boost their self-confidence.

In hospitals, massage has been used to ease pain and discomfort as well as being of benefit to people who are bedridden, since the flow of blood to the muscles is stimulated. It has also been used for those who have suffered a heart attack and has helped their recovery. A more recent development has been the use of massage for cancer patients who are suffering from the after-effects of treatment, such as chemotherapy, as well as the discomfort the disease itself causes. Indeed, there are few conditions when it is not recommended. However, it should not be used when people are suffering from inflammation of the veins (phlebitis), varicose veins, thrombosis (clots in the blood) or if they have a raised temperature such as occurs during a fever. It is then advisable to contact a doctor before using massage. Doctors may be able to recommend a qualified therapist, a health centre may be able to help or contact can be made with the relevant professional body.

It is quite usual nowadays for a masseur or masseuse to combine treatment with the use of other methods, such as aromatherapy, acupuncture or reflexology. Massage can be divided into four basic forms, and these are known as *percussion* (also known as drumming); *friction* (also called pressure); *effleurage* (also called stroking) and *petrissage* (also called kneading). These four methods can be practised alone or in combination for maximum benefit to the patient. Massage is a therapy in which both parties derive an overall feeling of wellbeing— the therapist by the skilful use of the hands to impart the relaxation, and the patient through the therapy being administered.

Percussion is also called tapotement, which is derived from *tapoter*, a French word that means 'to drum', as of the fingers on a surface. As would be expected from its name, percussion is generally done with the edge of the hand with a quick, chopping movement, although the strokes are not hard. This type of movement would be used on places like the buttocks, thighs, waist or shoulders where there is a wide expanse of flesh.

Friction is often used on dancers and athletes who experience problems with damaged ligaments or tendons. This is because the flow of blood is stimulated and the movement of joints is improved. Friction can be performed with the base of the hand, some fingers or the upper part of the thumb. It is not advisable to use this method on parts of the body that have been injured in some way, for example where there is bruising.

Effleurage is performed in a slow, controlled manner using both hands together with a small space between the thumbs. If the therapist wishes to use only light pressure he or she will use the palms of the hands or the tips of the fingers, whilst for increased pressure the knuckles or thumbs will be used.

Petrissage employs a kneading action on parts of a muscle. As the therapist works across each section, an area of flesh is grasped and squeezed, and this action stimulates the flow of blood and enables tensed muscles to relax. People such as athletes can have an accumulation of lactic acid in certain muscles, and this is why cramp occurs. Parts of the body on which this method is practised are along the stomach and around the waist.

A session may be undertaken in the patient's home, or he or she can attend the masseur or masseuse at a clinic. At each session the client will undress, leaving only pants or briefs on, and will lie on a firm, comfortable surface, such as a table that is designed especially for massage. The massage that follows normally lasts from 20 minutes to one hour. Women in labour have found that the pain experienced during childbirth can be eased if massage is performed on the buttocks and back. The massage eases the build-up of tension in the muscles, encouraging relaxation and easing of labour pains. It is said to be more effective on women who had previously experienced the benefits and reassurance of massage.

For anyone who is competent and wishes to provide some simple massage for a partner, there are some basic rules to follow. The room should be warm and peaceful. The surface on which the person lies is quite comfortable but firm. A futon (a quilted Japanese mattress) can be used, and to relieve the upper part of the body from any possible discomfort, a pillow should be placed underneath the torso. Any pressure that may be exerted on the feet can be dispelled by the use of a rolled-up towel or similar placed beneath the ankles. Both people should be relaxed, and to this end soft music can be played. All the movements of the hand should be of a continuous nature. It is suggested that the recipient always has one hand of the masseur or masseuse placed on him or her. Vegetable oil (about one teaspoonful) is suitable but should not be poured straight on to the person. It should be spread over the hands by rubbing, which will also warm it sufficiently for use. Should the masseur or masseuse get out of breath, he or she should stop for a rest, all the while retaining a hand on the person.

Massage of the head and face begins with the forehead, which should be massaged using the thumbs. This is done by stroking them outwards from the centre across the forehead. This can also be repeated for the cheeks. The jawline can then be squeezed along its full extent using the thumb and forefinger in a circular motion.

The head can be massaged by all the fingers using a circular motion. Whilst the person's head is being supported at the side, the muscles in the neck can be gently massaged, commencing at the top and moving downwards. To exercise the upper chest or pectoral muscles, move the base of the hands from the sternum (breastbone) outwards across these muscles. Both hands can be used to work upwards and also across the stomach area. Once the hands have moved across so that they are under the person's waist, raise the body slightly, thus stretching it. Another technique for the abdominal area is to glide the hands across but moving in opposite ways. The arm can be massaged by the fingers and thumb and then the fingers can be pressed and gently pulled, with the wrist being held at all times.

Effleurage (as described previously) can be used on the upper leg as far up as the hip on the outside of the leg. Once the person is lying face downwards (with support under the chest), continue to use effleurage movements on the back of the lower leg. Continue as before but work on the upper leg, avoiding the knee. The muscles in the buttocks can be worked upon with both hands to squeeze but making sure that the hands are moving in opposite ways. The foot will benefit from massage using the thumb in small circular movements. For a person suffering from stress or being 'on edge' at the end of a day's work, a back massage can help to ease these problems. With the hands in the position for using effleurage, start the movements at the lowest part of the back and work up and then sideways to the shoulders. The pressure used should be kept up, but as soon as the hands move downwards it should be released. This should be repeated so that all of the back is massaged. Next, using the palms of both hands, work on the top of the shoulder by moving the hands in opposite directions. If the right shoulder is being massaged, the person's head should be turned to the left. The area beside the spine can be massaged, although one should avoid the spinal column. Using both thumbs, one on each side of the spine itself, massage this area by pressing gently in a circle.

Massage has a wide range of uses for a variety of disorders. Its strengths lie in the easing of strain and tension and inducing relaxation and serenity, plus the physical contact of the therapist. Although doctors make use of this therapy in conjunction with orthodox medicine, it is not to be regarded as a cure for diseases in itself and serious problems could occur if this were the case.

Quick Guide to
Symptoms and Possible Causes

sudden or severe abdominal pain

Possible cause:

appendicitis

cholecystitis

colic

colitis

Crohn's disease

diverticular disease – diverticulitis

ectopic pregnancy

gallstones

ileitis

intestinal obstruction and intussusception

liver abscess

ovarian cyst (ruptured)

pancreas cancer

pancreatitis

peritonitis

porphyria

behavioural changes, dementia, psychological disturbance or disorder

Possible cause:

alcoholism

Alzheimer's disease

brain tumour

catalepsy

catatonia

concussion

Cushing's syndrome

delirium

drug abuse

epilepsy – temporal lobe epilepsy

head injury

Huntington's chorea
myxoedema
narcolepsy
porphyria
rabies
Reye's syndrome (stroke)
syphilis (transient ischaemic attack)

bleeding from the rectum, blood in faeces, pain
Possible cause:
anal fissure
cirrhosis of the liver
colitis
constipation
dysentery
gastric erosion
haemorrhoids
hepatoma
Polyarteritis nodosa
rectal abscess
rectal prolapse or rectocele
rectal tumour
small intestine tumour
stomach cancer
stomach ulcer
thrombocytopaenia

abnormal vaginal bleeding
Possible cause:
Abruptio placentae (pregnancy)
ectopic pregnancy
endometriosis
fibroid

pelvic inflammatory disease
Placenta praevia (pregnancy)
uterine cancer
vaginal cancer

unexplained or sudden bleeding
Possible cause:
AIDS
bone fracture
cirrhosis of the liver
haemophilia
haemorrhage
leukaemia
radiation sickness
subconjunctival haemorrhage (eye)
thrombocytopaenia

breathlessness, wheezing, breathing difficulty
Possible cause:
allergy
asbestosis
asthma
emphysema
hay fever

chest pain
Possible cause:
aneurysm
Angina pectoris
aortic valve disease
atrial fibrillation
coronary artery disease
coronary thrombosis (heart attack)

heartburn
pericarditis
pleurisy
pneumothorax
pulmonary embolism
pulmonary hypertension
pulmonary valve stenosis

chest pain with breathlessness, breathing difficulty, cough
Possible cause:
Angina pectoris
aortic valve disease
asbestosis
atrial fibrillation
bronchiolitis
cardiomyopathy
emphysema
mesothelioma
pericarditis
pneumoconiosis
silicosis
tapeworms

convulsions (fits)
Possible cause:
asphyxia
brain tumour
eclampsia of pregnancy
epilepsy
fever – and any infections which cause fever
head injury
meningitis
Reye's syndrome

pulmonary hypertension
Roseola infantum

abnormal vaginal discharge
Possible cause:
AIDS
fibroid in uterus
gonorrhoea
non-specific urethritis
ovarian cyst
pelvic inflammatory disease
Reiter's syndrome
uterine cancer
vaginitis

symptoms of ear disorder e.g. discharge, pain, ringing in ears (tinnitus), vertigo, nausea, vomiting, deafness
Possible cause:
deafness
labyrinthitis
Menière's disease
Otitis externa
Otitis media
otosclerosis
ruptured eardrum

fluid retention causing swelling (oedema)
Possible cause:
adult respiratory distress syndrome
allergy
anaphylactic shock
aneurysm
cardiomyopathy

cirrhosis of the liver
eclampsia of pregnancy
glomerulonephritis
haemolytic disease of the newborn
hepatitis
hepatoma
hydrocephalus
kidney failure
liver cancer
nephrotic syndrome
Polyarteritis nodosa
pre-eclampsia of pregnancy
pulmonary oedema
pulmonary valve stenosis
trichinosis

**gastro-intestinal symptoms – e.g. nausea, vomiting, diarrhoea,
abdominal pains, loss of appetite and weight, abnormal
stools, fever**
Possible cause:
ancyclostomiasis
Addison's disease
cholera
cirrhosis of the liver
coeliac disease
diverticular disease – diverticulosis
duodenal ulcer
fascioliasis
food poisoning
gastritis
gastroenteritis
giardiasis
irritable bowel syndrome

Lassa fever
ovarian tumour
Polyarteritis nodosa
roundworms
sprue
stomach ulcer
tapeworms

**headache possibly with other symptoms, e.g. numbness or
weakness, nausea and vomiting, confusion, vision disturbance**
Possible cause:
aneurysm
brain abscess
brain tumour
carbon monoxide poisoning
concussion encephalitis
glaucoma
head injury
heatstroke
hypertension
meningitis
migraine
temporal arteritis
sinusitis
subarachnoid haemorrhage
subdural haemorrhage

**symptoms of hormonal disorders – unexplained weight gain or
loss, gastro-intestinal upset, menstrual changes, unusual
growth of body hair, retarded or accelerated growth,
swelling, palpitations, anxiety**
Possible cause:
Addison's disease

Cushing's syndrome
Grave's disease
hyperthyroidism
myxoedema
ovarian tumour
phaeochromocytoma
thyroid gland tumour

inflammation of eyes or eyelids e.g. reddening, itching, pain, discharge
Possible cause:
blepharitis
conjunctivitis
corneal foreign body
entropion
iritis
keratitis
ptosis
scleritis
stye
subconjunctival haemorrhage

influenza-like symptoms e.g. headache, chills, shivering, fever, aches and pains, malaise, sore throat, swollen glands.
Possible cause:
AIDS
bronchitis
brucellosis
cat scratch fever
croup
dengue
diphtheria
glandular fever

Hodgkin's disease
influenza
Kawasaki disease
Lassa fever
Legionnaire's disease
leptospirosis
lung abscess
malaria
mumps
pneumonia
psittacosis
Q fever
sandfly fever
sinusitis
tonsillitis
toxocariasis
toxoplasmosis
tuberculosis
whooping cough

kidney symptoms; including pain in the lower back or abdomen, fever, blood or pus in urine, nausea, vomiting, chills, malaise, headache, fatigue, change in amount of urine passed, oedema and swelling
Possible cause:
glomerulonephritis
hypernephroma
kidney failure
kidney stones
myeloma
nephrotic syndrome
Polyarteritis nodosa
polycystic disease of the kidney

pyelitis
Reiter's syndrome
renal carbuncle
renal tuberculosis
scleroderma
systemic Lupus erythematosus
Wilm's tumour

symptoms of liver disorder; jaundice, loss of appetite and weight, fluid retention, fatigue, anaemia, dark coloured urine, digestive upset, itching skin
Possible cause:
cirrhosis of the liver
fascioliasis
hepatitis
hepatoma
leptospirosis
liver abscess
liver cancer
lymphoma
schistosomiasis
tapeworms
thalassaemia

symptoms of lung infection or inflammation; including cough with sputum or blood, chest pain, breathlessness, breathing difficulty, fever, chills, malaise
Possible cause:
asbestosis
bronchiectasis
bronchitis
chronic bronchitis
emphysema

Legionnaire's disease
lung abscess
lung cancer
pleurisy
pneumoconiosis
pneumonia
psittacosis
pulmonary oedema
Q fever
silicosis
tuberculosis

**mass or lump, including swollen glands, which can be felt
    externally**
Possible cause:
AIDS (glands)
boil (skin)
breast abscess
breast cancer
cat scratch fever (glands)
cirrhosis of liver
corns
diphtheria (glands in neck)
Ewing's sarcoma (bones)
glandular fever (glands in neck, armpits, groin)
Grave's disease (neck)
haemorrhoids (piles)
hepatoma (liver – abdomen)
hernia (abdomen, groin)
Hodgkin's disease (all glands)
hyperthyroidism (thyroid – neck)
ileitis (abdomen)
intestinal obstruction

Kaposi's sarcoma (feet, ankles, hands, arms, lymph glands)
Kawasaki disease (neck glands)
laryngeal cancer (lymph glands in neck)
leukaemia (lymph glands, spleen, liver)
lipoma (skin)
listeriosis (lymph glands)
liver abscess (abdomen)
liver cancer (abdomen)
lymphoma
mastitis (breast)
mumps (salivary glands in face, neck)
oesophageal cancer
osteosarcoma (bones, especially leg or arm)
ovarian tumour (abdomen)
pharyngitis (throat)
pyloric stenosis (stomach)
rectal abscess (rectum)
rectal prolapse (rectum)
rectal tumour (rectum)
salivary gland enlargement (mouth, neck)
sporotrichosis (skin)
stomach cancer
syphilis (lymph glands)
thyroid gland tumour (neck)
tonsillitis (neck, throat)
tooth abscess (face)
toxoplasmosis (lymph glands)

abnormal involuntary muscular twitches or spasms
Possible cause:
cerebral palsy
convulsions
epilepsy

Huntington's chorea
multiple sclerosis
Parkinson's disease

***nerve pain*; pain along the course of a nerve**
Possible cause:
Bell's palsy (face)
carpal tunnel syndrome (hands, arms)
neuralgia
neuritis
sciatica
shingles

**numbness or weakness, tingling, unsteadiness, paralysis, speech
   disorder, confusion**
Possible cause:
Bell's palsy (facial muscles)
brain compression
carpal tunnel syndrome (fingers, hands, arms)
cerebral palsy
Friedreich's ataxia
Guillain-Barré syndrome
Huntington's chorea
multiple sclerosis
muscular dystrophy
Myasthenia gravis
Paget's disease of bone
Parkinson's disease
Polyarteritis nodosa
polymyositis
ptosis
spondylosis
stroke

syphilis
transient ischaemic attack

pain, stiffness and inflammation around a joint with heat, swelling and, possibly, other symptoms such as fever, malaise etc.
Possible cause:
bursitis
dislocation
Ewing's sarcoma
frozen shoulder
gout
Legg-Calvé Perthes disease
Osgood-Schlatter's disease (knee)
osteoarthritis
psoriasis (psoriatic arthritis)
rheumatic fever
rheumatoid arthritis
scleroderma
Still's disease
systemic Lupus erythematosus
tendinitis

pain in the back with stiffness
Possible cause:
ankylosing spondylitis
bone fracture
osteoarthritis
osteoporosis
Paget's disease of bone
Polymyalgia rheumatica
prolapsed intervertebral disc
spondylosis
Still's disease

pains in the legs
Possible cause:
atherosclerosis
Buerger's disease
thromboembolism
thrombophlebitis
thrombosis (deep vein)
varicose veins

respiratory distress, e.g. breathing difficulty, breathlessness, cyanosis (blue tinge to skin), rapid, laboured breathing, chest pain, raised heartbeat rate.
Possible cause:
adult respiratory distress syndrome
anaphylactic shock
asphyxia
asthma (severe attack)
bronchiolitis
croup (severe attack)
diphtheria
pneumothorax (severe)
pulmonary oedema
shock

skin lesions or ulcers; possibly with e.g. fever, malaise, aches and pains, chills, headache
Possible cause:
agranulocytosis
AIDS
athlete's foot
boil or furuncle
Buerger's disease
burns and scalds

candidiasis (thrush)
chilblain
cold sores
corns and bunions
dermatitis
diabetes mellitus
eczema
erythema
erythroderma
erythromelalgia
frostbite
Granuloma annulare
hand, foot and mouth disease
Herpes simplex infection
icthyosis
impetigo
Kaposi's sarcoma
keratosis
Lupus erythematosus
melanoma
pemphigus
psoriasis
Raynaud's disease
Reiter's syndrome
ringworm
rodent ulcer
scabies
scleroderma
shingles
skin cancer
sporotrichosis
syphilis
thalassaemia

varicose veins
warts
yaws

skin rash; with or without accompanying symptoms of fever, malaise, chills, aches and pains, headache
Possible cause:
allergy
anaphylactic shock
chicken pox
German measles
Lassa fever
Lupus erythematosus
rosacea
Roseola infantum
scarlet fever
systemic Lupus erythematosus
thrombocytopaenia

severe or persistent sore throat, hoarseness, voice changes
Possible cause:
diphtheria
glandular fever
laryngeal cancer
laryngitis
pharyngitis
scarlet fever
tonsillitis

thirst
Possible cause:
Diabetes insipidus
Diabetes mellitus

vision disturbance or loss of vision
Possible cause:
brain tumour
cataract
glaucoma
Grave's disease
head injury
hydrocephalus
iritis
migraine
phaeochromocytoma
polycythaemia
retinal detachment
senile macular degeneration
stroke
tapeworms
thromboembolism
toxoplasmosis
transient ischaemic attack
trichinosis

vomiting
Possible cause:
Hyperemus gravidarum (rare condition of pregnancy)
pyloric stenosis

vomiting of blood
Possible cause:
gastric erosion
gastritis
stomach cancer
yellow fever (tropical disease)

urinary tract symptoms; urinary frequency, pain on passing urine, blood in urine

Possible cause:

bladder stones

bladder tumour

cystitis

fistula (urinary)

glomerulonephritis

gonorrhoea

hypernephroma

non-specific urethritis

ovarian cyst

prostate gland cancer

prostate gland enlargement

schistosomiasis (tropical disease)

urethra, stricture of

vaginal cancer